MONGERS IN HEAVEN

Sexual Tourism and HIV Risk in Costa Rica and in the United States

Jacobo Schifter-Sikora

University Press of America,® Inc.
Lanham · Boulder · New York · Toronto · Plymouth, UK

4501 Forbes Boulevard
Suite 200
Lanham, Maryland 20706
UPA Acquisitions Department (301) 459-3366

Estover Road
Plymouth PL6 7PY
United Kingdom

Printed in the United States of America
British Library Cataloging in Publication Information Available

Library of Congress Control Number: 2006931836
ISBN-13: 978-0-7618-3597-4 (paperback : alk. paper)
ISBN-10: 0-7618-3597-0 (paperback : alk. paper)

™ The paper used in this publication meets the minimum requirements of American National Standard for Information Sciences—Permanence of Paper for Printed Library Materials, ANSI Z39.48—1984

Contents

Methodology

In a talk given at the Albany campus of Massey University of New Zealand on the epistemology of research, Chris Ryan and C. Michael Martin (2000), authors of *Sex Tourism: Marginal People and Liminalities,* [1] provided a metaphor likening research truths to an onion. In their study of prostitution in Thailand, they found that women involved in the industry of sexual tourism had different answers to questions posed by different people in different circumstances. They described this as being like a sheet of an onion, which has its own truth, and its own logic that changes each time you peel it. They postulate that, as sex researchers, we confront partial truths. The truth lies in the whole onion rather than at a "core" or at one single layer.

Sexual work aims to please others and offers a theatre where fantasy and reality intermingle. This is the reason why sex researchers, who enter a brothel, nightclub or massage sauna, will receive a variant representation, generally the type of information they themselves want to hear. "Are you doing STI prevention?" our ethnographer asks a prostitute. "Yes, we are all concerned here and use condoms all the time," she responds. Yet, later she charges a client double to perform sex without a condom.

If the people who work in the sexual industry know that researchers belong to a nongovernmental or private organization in the health prevention field, they will probably say when questioned that safe sex is generally practiced, that the consumption of drugs is low or nonexistent, and that they work inside the industry because of harsh economic difficulties. Although we found other realities in our 2000 survey with sex workers, it is very probable that most of them underreported the amount of unsafe sex, drug consumption and misrepresented their reasons for engaging in sex work.

We did not find in our 2000 Survey a total commitment to safe sex. As a matter of fact, unsafe sex was high. Nevertheless, it is to be expected that if we factor in the underreporting –especially with regard to condom and drug use– the risk index would have been much higher.

Information–gathering and illegality

In Costa Rica, sex work is legal and the country has a strong tradition of tolerance toward prostitution. In 1894, the first laws *(Ley de Profilaxis Venérea and Reglamento de Prostitución)* were enacted to regulate and control the activity under the rationale that it was important for guaranteeing "hygiene and public morals." From then on, sex workers were subjected to a weekly medical check–up in order to detect sexually–transmitted diseases (STD's). Prostitutes had to register with the police and those who failed to do so, could be sentenced to a maximum of 10 days in prison. Women who were infected were forbidden to work and were subject to longer prison terms. Sex workers were prohibited from living 200 meters from schools and in cases of scandalous behavior, were expelled from their neighborhoods. Sex workers were listed in the public registry and could only be removed if they were married or had proof of a "respectable job." In the 1943–1944 Penal Code, supervision of sex workers was handed to social workers. This proved to be problematic since sex workers were able to evade these officials.In the present Penal Code of 1970, it is again the Ministry of Health that is responsible for periodically testing registered sex workers. Those who do not comply are subject to arrest by the police. [2]

The Costa Rican Penal Code of 1894 was emulated by the Netherlands in its 1911 Code that legalized prostitution. The Dutch penal code defined the broader context for prostitution laws and regulations in their colonies: brothels were banned throughout the kingdom and the active promotion of prostitution, as in Costa Rica, was criminalized. Nevertheless, prostitution was considered a necessary social evil, and sex work itself was not criminalized, allowing some forms of tolerance of sex work and the legal existence of the social category of the prostitute. In Dutch colonies such as Curazao and Aruba, there was greater tolerance than in the Netherlands, and brothels –like the famous Campo Alegre– were set up. This led to government intervention in and regulation of prostitution and provided an active role for the police in guaranteeing that sex workers were "free of disease." Thus, the states that legalized prostitution and took it upon themselves to protect "society from prostitution's evil influence," became directly involved in the sex trade. [3]

Although prostitution is legal in Costa Rica, pimping[4] (*proxenetismo*) is not. Many practices can be considered pimping and thus be illegal. According to a strict reading of this law, an individual who owns a nightclub that promotes prostitution can be prosecuted for pimping. Massage parlors, hotels that cater to prostitutes, and bars with private rooms, can all be legally prosecuted as well. Furthermore, the manner in which sex workers are paid can determine what is considered legal and illegal. Dildoman, for example, explains to other sex tourists that Art y Sauna, a massage parlor, was closed by a "technical" interpretation of the Law: Since the receptionist would "collect all the money from the client and then pay the '*chicas*' the authorities considered that as pimping."[5]

In addition to pimping, establishments and individuals are often prosecuted for other reasons. The police and the Ministry of Health may crack down on places that employ HIV–positive sex workers and illegal residents, detain American tourists who do not have their papers at hand and imprison owner and managers if there is a minor on the premises. This vulnerability to police harassment and blackmail is one of the worst fears among those involved in the sex industry.

The first warning usually comes from newspaper articles. A.M., a newspaper, tells mongers that the Ministry of Health will make sure that the massage parlors are not being used for prostitution and that it will take measures to "avoid the camouflage of places of prostitution that function under the name of massage parlors."[6] A few days later, the police raid the Massage Parlors and their clients are imprisoned. In other circumstances, the arrival of a questionable individual is the trigger. Jeff99 –for example– is aware of the danger that "Easy", a sex tourist, is in San José. This man is looked for the police for "his Sex Wax scam he perpetrated last November." Since he is in town he thinks, "new raids are to be expected this week." Mongers or sex tourists –he believes– will pay collective punishment. "The smart thing to do" he adds "is to remember that Easy is a long time member of this Forum" and to "carry your passports this week if you are in town, especially if you're in the vicinity of Mr. Easy. Easy arrives on June 28th. Be on the lookout. Be careful out there gentlemen."[7]

The manner these mongers act reminds us of the homosexual harassment in the 1970's. In that decade, the police used to have periodic raids on gay bars. Once the police were spotted, bar owners would turn on a red light to warn their customers. Gay couples immediately stopped dancing with each other and ran to the exit doors. Twenty years later, heterosexual American males are the ones who fear persecution from the police.

Romulus, for example, is coming to town and wants to know if there have been any raids recently. If the answer is affirmative, he asks other mongers what to do: "Do you run for the elevators or exit doors? How about stairways or inside the kitchen downstairs?"[8]

Paco Loco, another sex tourist, does not understand why there are raids if prostitution is legal in Costa Rica.[9] Romulus explains to him that the harassment is "irrational" and that American tourists are not immunized to police raids.[10] The Government wants, for its part, to show that "they are fighting prostitution."[11]

There is an ongoing debate among experts on how the illegality of sex work affects both the sex tourist and the sex worker. Ryan and Hall in their work on Southeast Asia view sex tourism as an interaction between two groups of equally positioned yet marginalized people –tourists and prostitutes. They identify three main features common to tourists and sex workers. The first one is the power of dressing, the second involves sensuality or undressing; and the third, the formation of particular spatial communities. The authors argue that tourists and prostitutes both occupy a position of power, the "working girl exercises the power to earn cash; the tourist exercises power due to the possession of money."[12] Conversely, Kempadoo, in her studies of sex tourism in the Caribbean, views sexual tourists as part of a dominating culture treated with respect by the country's police and by everyone in the sex industry. Sex tourists, mostly white, are seen as members of a distinguished and powerful group that provides work for millions of people. She believes the "liminal model" does not apply to the Caribbean:

> *It is however not an explanation that serves the Caribbean well. The tourist as a marginal person is a questionable notion in the Caribbean context, given the extreme dominance of tourism in the region and the kinds of preferential treatment that tourists receive. Caribbean governments are subservient to the global economy and the foreign exchange brought in by tourists, and a person holding a greenback or Euro commands service and deference.*[13]

The Costa Rican case seems to follow more Ryan and Hall's model of liminality. Sex tourists are afraid of the police and with good reasons. Examples of this are a monger who had to dress as a Chef in a hotel to avoid being taken to prison; another who hid in the garbage to avoid the police; a third jumped over a fence, and broke his leg to avoid being caught inside a brothel. Contrary to the experience in the Caribbean where being white is a historical prerogative, it is not a passport to exercise power in Costa Rica. The Catholic Church has a much stronger influence in Costa Rican politics (It is the State Religion) than the protestant churches in the English Caribbean. Mongers[14] in Costa Rica, may be more apprehensive about publicly participating in the sex trade and do not feel so powerful as to do whatever they wish with regard to sex workers. They know that in case of getting involved with minors, they might land in jail.

The vulnerable sexual industry implies that sex researchers are not welcomed and that none of the club owners are to volunteer information that could eventually put them in prison. Sex workers themselves are afraid of those whose motivations are not sexual. If the interviewer turns out to be a journalist or a policeman and gathers evidence that sex is being performed on the premises, the place can be closed down and foreign sex workers can be deported. In the case where the sex worker is a mother, she can lose custody over her children.

Nevertheless, with the present situation it is impossible to tell who is a researcher and who is an undercover agent and anyone who asks too many questions might be either one of them. We get evidence of the sex industry's fear from one of the sex forums when sex tourists discuss over an invitation by a Chicago journalist to do a piece on them. King Kosta thinks this is "a very lousy idea ... please."[15] Dboy agrees with him and considers the thought of helping write such an article something "ridiculous."[16] Tman asks others who might consider to participate: "Do we really need to parade around the fun things we do in the dark to everyone in the world . . . including wives, mothers and Ch*ldren? Dont think so." (sic) An article such as the one proposed is, in his opinion, a "public scrutiny and knowledge that bring out the witch hunts and double standards of government types to limit the personal freedoms of pleasure seekers." Journalists and researchers only want "sensationalism and anything 'shocking' to sell newspapers, mags or get eyes on TV in Jerry Springer –like fashion." For these reasons he suggests that "The last thing I want to see is some of my favorite Ticas brought into the States, paraded on Springer and other like shows, and fighting on live TV over whether they both slept with me or not." Finally, his recommendation is fierce: "I encourage you guys NOT to spill the beans . . . ."[17]

Monger's fear makes it difficult to gain accessibility to the world of Costa Rican prostitution. The RAPID ASSESSMENT or RAP[18] is a good tool to counteract the tendency to lie since it approaches this universe from different angles and different sources of information. By using triangulation it lessens the distortions expected from a community that is liminal, hidden and secretive, and wants to remain as invisible as possible. Despite our efforts, the RAP is a short intervention that lasts a couple of months and aims at gathering as much information as possible. The number of informants, focus groups, ethnographic observations and in–depth interviews are kept small.

The surveys

In 1997 and in 2000 ILPES (The Latin American Health and Prevention Institute) carried out a Survey funded by USAID/PASMO on Central American and Costa Rican sex workers. The objective of the research was to study the use of condoms and related factors. The Surveys provided invaluable information on sex workers from brothels, nightclubs, massage parlors and from street workers. It did not include sex workers who work at the major hotels that cater to American tourists. Nevertheless, 75% of sex tourists in the poll taken at www.costaricaticas.com, a sex forum, also cater to the places studied in the ILPES' surveys.[19]

The sample size was established according to time and economic constraints. It was agreed to have a sample of 400 female sex workers both from the street and from brothels, bars or discos in San José, Costa Rica.

An estimate was made of the number of sex workers who work in the establishments and in the streets.[20] The random nature of the sample was established by the choice of hours for interviews.[21] Finally, 400 interviews were carried out at the different social centers in San José.[22]

Focus–group discussions

A sample of 10 sex workers were invited to participate in focus–group discussions held at ILPES in San José, Costa Rica. These were carried out on July 29, 2000 from 8 pm to 10:30 pm.[23] The discussions focused on participant's perception of the data gathered with regard to sexual risk–taking in association with substance use and possibilities of behavior change.[24]

In–depth interviews

A sub–sample of 20 sex workers was invited to take part in individual semi–structured in–depth interviews about their perceptions and behavior concerning psychoactive substance use and sexuality. These interviews had an average duration of one hour and were conducted in three nightclubs in San José, Costa Rica. Five interviewers participated during the month of September 2000.[25]

Another five interviewers (not the same ones conducting the focus–group interviews) received special training on how to respond constructively to possible sensitive information given by the participants and possible feelings of embarrassment and shame.[26]

Ethnographic observation

In 2000 two nightclubs were selected for ethnographic observation: Puro Placer and Elías [27]. Puro Placer is a club located near the Coca Cola Market in San José, Costa Rica. The area is part of San José's red–light district. The observation took place on March 24, 2000 and was conducted by two ethnographers, one male and one female. They spent five hours in this bar. Elite is a similar club located in Paseo Colón, a more commercial section in the city of San José. The same ethnographers conducted the observation during May 26, 2000 from 10:30 pm to 1 o'clock in the morning.

The nightclubs have approximately from 20 to 40 female dancers and a clientele of approximately 100 to 200 men per night. The bars are meeting places for prostitutes and their clients who, after several drinks, retire to nearby motels, private apartments or houses. The main activity in both places is dancing and drinking. [28]

2004 RAP

To update the data, another RAP was conducted in 2004, during the months of September, October and November. This time the emphasis was placed on sex workers who cater to American clients and on the clients themselves. The following interventions took place:

- Mapping of the most important sexual establishments in San José and in Jaco Beach that cater to American tourists.
- A study on sex forums and websites that promote sexual tourism to Costa Rica in Internet. [29]
- In–depth interviews with 10 sex workers at Hotel Del Buey and Tea Amargo.
- Ethnographic observation in Hotel Del Buey and Tea Amargo
- In–depth interviews with 15 waiters and taxi drivers.
- Ethnographic observation in massage parlors and nightclubs.
- Two focus–groups with 10 sex workers.
- In–depth interviews with 10 sex workers in Tango India nightclub.
- Five in–depth interviews with Ministry of Health officers.

Quotes

We opted to leave the posts from the Internet just as they are found, with typos, misspellings and words in Spanish.

Background

In general terms, Costa Rica is definitely the nation with the highest rate of development in Central America. It has the best reputation on many levels to that of its neighbors [30]. With a long history of democracy, tolerance, republicanism and pacifism, Costa Rica offers a level of education, economic development and better standard of living than the other countries in the area. Since its origin as an independent nation, Costa Rica wanted to isolate itself from the social and political torment of its neighbors. For decades it was an oasis of relative tranquility and stability in the midst of a region torn by militarism and war, and played a fundamental role in the pacification process that spread through Central America beginning in the middle of the 80's. Since the 19th century, Costa Rican leaders have been concerned about how to capitalize on the social advantages of the country, whose attributes have become part of traditionally accepted mythology, illustrated in names describing Costa Rica as "the Switzerland of Central America" and the "Garden of Peace."

Having been part of the Spanish Empire for close to three centuries, Costa Rica gained its independence in 1821. At the time of initial contact with the European colonizers, the indigenous population of what is now Costa Rica did not exceed 25,000 souls, making it one of the most sparsely populated regions of Central America. [31] During much of the Colonial period Roman Catholicism enjoyed a monopoly over the minds and souls of the country's inhabitants, as it was the only religion tolerated by Costa Rica's Spanish rulers. [32] In the field of economics, the era of Spanish rule was characterized most notably by chronic poverty, with a lack of human resources and mineral wealth ensuring that there was little in the way of sustained growth. This placed the country in the same disadvantaged position as other regions in Latin American without mineral resources. Costa Rica attracted little immigration throughout the three centuries of Spanish domination. [33]

The country's peasant–based economy did establish sporadic links with the world market thanks to crops such as cocoa and tobacco. During the cocoa "boom" in the XVII Century, Black–enslaved labor was brought in from the Caribbean. Nevertheless, once the exports started to fall, these workers were freed and let to marry within the mostly white population. Both Indians and Blacks, as it happened in the rest of Latin America, saw intermarriage as an avenue for upward social mobility. "Whitening" became part of the sexual culture as it provided the key to obtain better jobs and access to the dominant Spanish society. [34]

With the advent of widespread coffee cultivation in the mid–nineteenth century, Costa Rica was integrated into the global chain of commodity production and consumption on a more permanent basis. Costa Rica for one had some of the fastest growth and development in Latin American during the nineteenth century. In the post–World War II period, government policies of import substitution galvanized the industrial sector while attracting large numbers of European immigrants, whose presence contributed in turn to an expansion of the country's ethnic and religious composition. At present, roughly 85 percent of Costa Rica's population calls itself Roman Catholic, while the rest self–identify with a range of Protestant and non–Christian religions. The population is mostly white and mestizo, with the exception of those descendants of Jamaican immigrants who came in the late 19th Century to work in the banana plantations and a small native aboriginal population.

The country today has a higher standard of living than many Latin American nations. Its per capita income is six times larger than Nicaragua, three times larger than Bolivia's and two times larger than the Dominican Republic's. Costa Rica has one of the highest literacy percentage rates in Latin America, one of the lowest children's mortality rates per 100,000 people and one of the highest life expectancies in the world.[35]

Despite the undoubted contribution made by coffee to Costa Rica's economic growth, it also served to make the country extremely vulnerable to the boom and bust cycle of the world commodity market. Economic recessions led to the famous military interventions during the 1900s in numerous Latin American republics such as Mexico and Peru. This was not true of Costa Rica, where the existence of an agricultural frontier zone until roughly the middle of the twentieth century contributed to the emergence of a large middle class and to the establishment of a democratic tradition that was interrupted only twice in this century. In 1948, following the second of these interruptions, Costa Rica's government abolished its armed forces.

In this way, the country was able to weave a social fabric where polarization and anomie were never permitted to reach the levels seen in other parts of Latin America, where military dictatorship was the rule rather than the exception. The program of social reform first embarked upon by the government of Calderón Guardia in the 1940s, subsequently deepened and strengthened by José Figueres Ferrer's Social Democratic Party, laid the groundwork for a welfare state that put Costa Rica on par with First World countries in such areas as literary and health. Notwithstanding the good achievements in health and social security, approximately one–third of Costa Rica's population lives bellow the poverty line. The country shares problems with the rest of the region such as unemployment, urban decay, increasing crime rates, and drugs.

Sexual culture

When the American sexual tourist writes that Costa Rican sex workers act "irrationally" or "lie compulsively", there is a hermeneutic problem. Latin American sexual culture is different from her Anglo–Saxon counterpart and it can be misunderstood by those who ignore its history. First, we need to take into account that Spain was able to dominate Latin America for three centuries without having to use a strong military force. Notwithstanding the imposition of high taxes and of prohibitions against developing local industries, there was little political armed resistance against Spain. The reason was simple. The Spanish Crown might have wished to exploit her American colonies, but in reality she was a declining power, unable to compete with England and with other European rivals, and incapable of supplying the New World with the needed industrial goods. She did not take advantage of such captive markets and instead of investing in her own development, the Spanish Crown squandered her wealth on European military interventions. [36]

Being unable to provide what in theory she declared as her monopoly, the Spanish Crown could not impose its will on the region. It learned to compromise and to look the other way both economically and politically. Despite the monopoly on manufactured goods, the local populations were left in practice to trade with the emerging powers. The same would happen in the political arena. Spain declared that the most important political posts had to be filled by "*Peninsulares*" or Spanish–born citizens. Nevertheless, the Crown was unable to pay for their salaries and started to sell these posts to those with money. In this way, many Latin American–born Spaniards or "*Mestizos*" (mixed Indian and Spanish) were able to purchase public office and acquire political power.

This created a culture of "I obey but do not comply." This meant that local authorities decided not to confront the system openly but –at the same time– did not follow the law. Since the Colonial power was so removed from the day–to–day affairs, so slow to respond because of its centralizing ideology, and so incapable of enforcing the enacted legislation, it became easier to ignore it. [37] The *mestizo*'s ability to exert influence on the Crown by refusing to implement any counterproductive legislation, lessened their need to break away from the Empire. The independence movements arose precisely when the Napoleonic Wars disrupted this system. This led to the Borbon's (The French side of the family) attempt to control Latin America by forbidding contraband and eradicating corruption in political offices. Only then did new Latin American elites decide to wage the wars of independence. [38]

The same dichotomy between theory and practice characterized the social. Latin America was taught a very radical form of Christian sexual ethics by a

Spanish Crown that emerged victorious after 800 hundred years of war against the infidels, i.e. the Muslims who had invaded the Spanish Peninsula. As the war dragged on, so did religious fanaticism, military chauvinism and a version of masculinity called "machismo." As Spain became more militaristic and "feudal", social minorities and women came to be more oppressed.[39] The war against the infidels culminated in 1492 when the Catholic Kings managed to launch the conquest of the New World as well as the expulsion of the Jews and the Muslims from Spain. The Colonization of the Americas would take place within a climate of religious fundamentalism and of social and ethnic intolerance. As Spain emerged victorious against her "internal" and "external" enemies in the Old World, she insisted in tightening her control over the New World. The feared Inquisition was transported to the Americas to oversee the minds and souls of the conquered populations.

Catholicism was imposed in the same manner as the export economy and political authoritarianism. People were to follow the new principles without having the right to question them. Jews and Protestants were forbidden to migrate to the Spanish colonies and the indigenous populations were forced to convert to Christianity. Heretics and false converts were put to death. The sexual ethics of Catholicism was strict: sex was acceptable only within marriage; divorce was outlawed; erotic pleasure was perceived as the devil's temptation. Prostitution and infidelity were severely punished. Children begotten outside marriage had no rights. Sodomites were burned at the stake.[40]

Notwithstanding the Catholic's position on sex, Latin America faced the same problems in the spiritual as in the economic realm: the impossibility of compliance. The region needed to develop through labor and labor was the main factor of development. Given the lack of immigration to the region, this could only take place through lax sexual mores, crossbreeding and high fertility. The countries that could increase the labor pool were the ones to develop faster. Thus, even as the Roman Catholic hierarchy in Colonial San José condemned divorce and fornication, it was pragmatic enough to recognize its own powerlessness to enforce these edicts. In the face of these contradictions, the Church became increasingly concerned with form rather than substance, while turning a blind eye to the burgeoning population of illegitimate children. Married men would set second houses for their mistresses and have as many children as possible.[41]

Given that the Catholic principles were not faithfully followed and that the Church itself unofficially accepted the particular sexual realities in the Colonies, there was no need to rebel. People learned to live with the contradictions between theory and practice. This is the historical "Compartmentalization" of Latin America. Catholic sexual prudishness survived its usefulness and the people's loyalty without having to be debated, questioned or abandoned. A new sexual ethic was developed: "Have sex but do not talk about it." People were let alone to live their sexualities without interference as long as the forbidden sexual practices were not made public. The population learned that as long as it was discreet, people would ignore sexual transgressions. This sexual ideology developed stronger from the periphery to the center. As economic resources dwindled among the poor and the marginal classes, the ideals of marriage, chastity and sexual control waned even further. Marriage became a mostly middle and upper class institution and cohabitation and sexual promiscuity were widespread.

As the country became wealthier after the 1950's, the nuclear family became the ideal sexual model. Young people were supposed to marry young and stay together for the rest of their lives. The high cost of living made it more difficult for men to keep more than one family and the second house became a relic of the past. The women's movement also started to demand more gender equal relationships and the abandonment of Latin machismo. [42]

US–Costa Rican relations

Tourists prefer to travel to friendly foreign countries were they are not subjected to hatred or disdain from the locals. After 9/11, Americans are more aware of where they are headed for their vacations. Today, they favor countries that are closer to home, Christian and not hostile to the US. There is no mystery then that Costa Rica has become one of the new favorite spots. In 2004, the number of tourists that traveled to Costa Rica rose by 25% and by another 20% in 2005. [43] American sex tourists are also on the rise and as we will see later, they find Costa Rica to be one of the friendliest places in Latin America.

This perception has historical roots. The US and Costa Rica share some important traditions which have set them apart from the more turbulent relations in the rest of the region. The Marines, for example, have never invaded the country, as has been the case in the rest of Central America and in the Caribbean. Costa Rica has economically and politically supported America during World War II, in all her regional and global conflicts, including the Cold War and the current struggle against Islamic fundamentalism. Furthermore, Costa Rica was one of the few Latin American countries that supported the war against Hussein in Iraq. This is not simply the result of America's bullying Costa Rica due to her overwhelming power as might have been the case with other nations in Latin America. San José has felt that their national interests have been closely linked to the American's since their independence and that both countries are "natural allies." This in turn has created a social and political atmosphere of true respect and liking toward American citizens.

One important reason for Costa Rica's close relation to the US is her "isolationist" policies with regard to Central America.[44] This means that she has refused to follow the other Central American countries' attempts to reunify the former Republic of Central America. Costa Rica distrusts Guatemala, the former capital of the Republic, and has fought against all her attempts to re–impose unification by force, which in practice meant endless wars. In this stand, Costa Rica has stood beside the United States, who has also opposed a possible Central American unification since this would neutralize her influence in the Isthmus. During all the Central American wars that had as their goal to impose a new Central America Republic, the US and Costa Rica have stood together as military allies. Since Costa Rica has had a weaker military force than the other countries in the region, the strategic dependence on the United States has been of great importance. After dissolving her armed forces in 1949, Costa Rica relies entirely for her independence on the Rio Treaty, and in practical terms, on the US. During the 1980's with the Sandinistas in power in Nicaragua, Costa Rica relied more than ever on the US for her sovereignty.[45]

Costa Rica's isolationist policies were a result of many factors. Firstly, Costa Rica is geo–politically distant from the rest of Central America. Its only common border is with Nicaragua, and much of its international trade during the Colonial Period was carried out through the Panamanian province of Chiriquí. This geographical separation has been aggravated by the awful conditions of communication in Central America. Secondly, the ethnic composition of the population is different from that of the rest of the Isthmus. With a predominantly homogeneous white population, Costa Rica has not been the victim of the cultural divisions of the other Central American countries. Finally, the economic development of Costa Rica, based on Spanish labor and not on the exploitation of the natives, produced a more egalitarian society. This created a more middle class society where extreme poverty is rare.[46] It also minimized illegal immigration to the United States and lessened resentment in both societies. Both economies suffer from waves of immigration of Central American refugees and illegal workers.

From 1898, onwards, the country was able to lay the foundation of a democratic, constitutional system. The Liberal period in Costa Rica, during the last two decades of the nineteenth century and the first three of the twentieth century, saw no dictatorships of the kind experienced in the rest of the Isthmus. In contrast to the Liberal governments of Rufino Barrios in Guatemala and José Santos Zelaya in Nicaragua, the Liberal regimes in Costa Rica were characterized by a respect for individual rights and the constitutional process. This adherence to a democratic system has led Costa Rican politicians to feel isolated in their Central American orbit and closer to the American sphere of influence.[47]

American investors did not cause the same conflicts in Costa Rica as they did in other Central American nations. Costa Rica took full advantage of these investors to carry out national projects. The construction of the Atlantic railroad, for example, was paid by the American Minor Keith, who would use the train to create its banana empire and his future United Fruit Company. Costa Rica, provided Keith with hundreds of thousands of vacant acres to plant the bananas, but she obtained in return a port that enabled her to trade and make millions out of coffee exports to the US and Europe. The country today relies on ecological tourism as her main source of foreign currency, an activity that does not create the antagonism of "maquilas" in the rest of Central America.

Another element which helped to reduce friction between the United States and Costa Rica was the responsible handling of foreign loans at various times. The United States had resorted to taking over the customs of a number of Caribbean and Central American countries, when these were unable to fulfill their financial obligations. From the United States standpoint, these interventions prevented creditors, mostly Europeans, from meddling in American affairs. But this was not the case with Costa Rica. Even during the difficult years of World War I, when the government experienced a considerable drop of income, the country met its obligations.[48]

America had such respect for Costa Rica's sovereignty that even in cases of turmoil such as during the Central American country's Civil War in 1948, the US Government decided against any military intervention. Washington let the Costa Ricans resolve their conflicts on their own, despite of fears that the Communist Party might control the streets of San José.[49]

When American sex tourists and Costa Rican sex workers walk the streets of San José, they might not be aware of the historical relationship between their respective countries. Nevertheless, both are reacting to a past that has been devoid of severe confrontations. This is not the same feeling American tourists experience when walking the streets of Guatemala, Nicaragua or El Salvador, where the people have grievances against past American invasions, past American support to dictatorships that killed hundreds of thousands of people or current American companies' policies that pay low salaries to Central American workers.

Notes

1. Chris Ryan and Michael Hall, *Sex Tourism and Liminalities,* Routledge: New York– London, 2001, p.xiv.

2. Asamblea Legislativa de Costa Rica, *Código de la niñez y la adolescencia.* Ley N° 7739. San José, Costa Rica, 1998.______________. "Código Penal", Ley N° 4573.

San José, Costa Rica, 1970.

3. Kamala Kempadoo, *Sexing the Caribbean. Gender, Race, and Sexual Labor*, Routledge: New York and London, 2004, ebook, p.1652.

4. Pimping: the act of a third party benefiting from the prostitution of another individual or group of individuals.

5. http://www.costaricaticas.com/phpbb2/viewtopic.php?t=1176

6. http://www.costaricaticas.com/phpbb2/viewtopic.php?t=1399

7. http://www.costaricaticas.com/phpbb2/viewtopic.php?t=2651

8. http://www.costaricaticas.com/phpbb2/viewtopic.php?t=1399

9. http://www.costaricaticas.com/phpbb2/viewtopic.php?t=2651

10. http://www.costaricaticas.com/phpbb2/viewtopic.php?t=2031

11. http://www.costaricaticas.com/phpbb2/viewtopic.php?t=2031

12. Chris Ryan and Michael Hall, *Sex Tourism and Liminalities*, Routledge, New York– London, 2001, p.4.

13. Kamala Kempadoo, *Sexing the Caribbean. Gender, Race and Sexual Labor*, London: Routledge, 2004, ebook, p. 2024

14. Mongers: name that refers to sex tourists

15. http://www.costaricaticas.com/phpbb2/viewtopic.php?t=1423

16. http://www.costaricaticas.com/phpbb2/viewtopic.php?t=1423

17. http://www.costaricaticas.com/phpbb2/viewtopic.php?t=1423

18. Sex– RAR Guide, The Rapid Assessment and Response Guide on Psychoactive Substance Use and Sexual Risk Behavior, Mental Health: Research and Evidence, Department of Mental Health and Substance Dependence, World Health Organization, Geneva, 2002.

19. http://www.costaricaticas.com/phpbb2/viewtopic.php?t=1863

20. The estimates cannot represent an exact number of sex workers since the women who frequent these places are not always the same, nor do they arrive with the same frequency. In addition, the opening hours of these places differ, and the number of sex workers can fluctuate due to the client's patterns of attendance.

21. Once an hour was randomly selected, the interviewer had to interview the first five sex workers that walked in the establishment. In the case of those who worked in the streets, different spaces and times were selected randomly and the interviewer had to select the sex worker who was present at that specific time.

22. In this case, the sampling procedure was applied with probability proportional to the size of the establishment (number of people visiting a given place–PPS). For this reason, each woman was weighed up in a proportionally inverse relation to the number of times she frequents the place. This variable was included in the questionnaire: "How many days a month do you attend these premises?"

23. The group was briefed on the purpose of the discussion, the background of the study, benefits to participants and others, the time it would take to take part in the discussion, steps taken to protect anonymity, how to access psycho–social support during and after the discussion, and whom to approach to discuss and explain details of the study. Participants were asked to put down a 'code–name' on the informed consent sheet instead of signing it personally. They were also handed out a copy of the informed consent sheet that did not specify their code name.

24. Two interviewers received special training on how to respond to potentially sensitive information given by the participants. They used participatory methodology to conduct the sessions. Focus group discussions were taped and transcribed. All tapes were erased after the conclusion of the study. There were no material inducements for participants, beyond free refreshments.

25. Participants were asked to put down their 'code–name' on the informed consent sheet instead of signing it personally. They were also given a copy of the informed consent sheet that did not specify their code name.

26. Interviews were recorded and transcribed following the strict safety procedures outlined above (including erasure of tapes after transcription, coding of names of other individuals mentioned in the course of the interview). There were no material inducements for participants, beyond the offer of free refreshments.

27. These are not their real names. All bar, hotel, night–club and Massage Parlor's names have been changed.

28. Confidentiality was maintained through the use of code names when writing field notes, storage of data in lockable filing cabinets, and limiting data–access to the research team.

29. We decided to leave the citations from the sex forums just as they were, without changing the spelling and the grammar.

30. Costa Rica, for example, has a reputation for being a safe and peaceful country with an educated population.

31. León Fernández, *Historia de Costa Rica,* San José: Imprenta Lehman, 1939.

32. James Backer, *La Iglesia y el sindicalismo en Costa Rica,* San José: Editorial Costa Rica, Second Edition, 1975.

33. Charles F. Denton, *Patterns of Costa Rican Politics,* The Allyn and Bacon Series in Latin American Politics. Boston: Allyn and Bacon, Inc., 1971.

34. León Fernández, *Historia de Costa Rica,* San José: Imprenta Lehman, 1939.

35. Jacobo Schifter, *The Construction of Latino Youth. Implications for the spread of HIV/AIDS,* New York: Haworth Press, 2000, p.8.

36. Hugh Thomas, *Rivers of Gold: The Rise of the Spanish Empire, from Columbus to Magellan,* New York: Radom House Publishing Group, 2004.

37. John R. Fisher, *Economic Aspects of Spanish Imperialism in America, 1492–1810,* Liverpool: Liverpool University Press, 1997.

38. Don Paul Abbott, *Rhetoric in the New World: Rhetorical Theory and Practice in Colonial Spanish America,* South Carolina: University of South Carolina Press, 1996.

39. Ann Twinam, Public Lives, *Private Secrets: Gender, Honor, Sexuality, and Illegitimacy in Colonial Spanish America,* Standford: Stanford University Press, 2001.

40. John Frederick Schwaller, Colin M. MacLachlan (Editor), William H. Beezley (Editor), *Church in Colonial Latin America,* Scholarly Resources, Inc., 2000.

41. Robert H. Jackson, *Race, Caste, and Status: Indians in Colonial Spanish America,* New Mexico: University of New Mexico Press, 1999.

42. Jacobo Schifter, *The Construction of Latino Youth. Implications for the spread of HIV/AIDS,* New York: Haworth Press, 2000, Chapters 6 and 7.

43. La Nacion, "*Aumento de turismo en 20%*" San Jose, Costa Rica, December 15, 2005, p.5A.

44. Chandler, P., Anderson, "Central American Policy of Non–Recognition." The American Journal of International Law, XIX (1925), 164–166.

45. Charles E. Chapma, "The Failure of Central American Union," The American Review of Reviews, LXV (July–December, 1922), 613–617.

46. Richard V. Salisbury, "*Costa Rican Relations with Central America, 1920–1936*," Unpublished Ph.D Dissertation, University of Kansas, 1970.

47. Kenneth J. Grieb, *The Myth of a Central American Dictator's League.* Journal of Latin American Studies 10 (November 1978), 329–45.

48. Suzanne O'Connor, *Costa Rica in the World Community of Nations, 1919–1939*, A Case Study in Latin American Internationalism, Unpublished Ph.D Dissertation, Loyola University, 1976.

49. Jacobo Schifter, *Las Alianzas Conflictivas.* San José. Editorial Libro Libre, 1984.

1. Is Costa Rica a new Thailand?

American Airlines Flight 971 from Miami to San José is jam–packed. More than 200 tourists, most of them American citizens, are headed to a country that was not very well known in the States until some years ago. Not only are there more than 12 daily flights from the United States to Costa Rica, but people have learned to identify the country on a map and to know at least somebody who has been or is headed here for a vacation.

If we were able to look inside the tourist's suitcases, we'd find the reasons for choosing this Central American country: snorkeling masks and flippers, scuba diving equipment, mountaineer's and riding equipment, and the one item no one can travel without: cameras. Every brochure about Costa Rica explains what to do: "Fly through the rain–forest canopy on a zip line? Go white–water rafting? Climb a volcano? Laze on a white–sand beach? Check out colorful marine life while snorkeling? Or try to hook one on a deep–sea fishing excursion?" Costa Rica –no doubt– offers plenty of pleasant choices like these, especially if you're interested in nature and outdoor activities. That's why so many people have chosen to come here: In the past decade, the number of visitors has quadrupled, and tourism has become a big part of the nation's economy.

To learn about tourist's fears we could also find in their purses and briefcases: allergy medicine, cold medicine, cough drops, headache medicine, Mycitracin or other salve for wounds, Insect repellant, After Bite (for relief of itching), Calamine lotion, Chigarid (for chigger bites), Tweezers, Magnifying glass (to spot splinters), Lip balm, Suntan lotion and anti–diarrhea medicine. Other items commonly found are: condoms, both male and female, Vaseline, and bottles of Viagra, Levitra and Cialis, as well as birth control pills and patches. Interestingly enough, some of the men's briefcases would also have plenty of small bottles of women's shampoos and conditioners, body lotions, mascara, nailbrushes, perfumes and make–up. The owners of these items are not gay or "Metrosexuals," but sixty –and seventy– year old grandfathers who are taking presents to "*novias*" or girlfriends.

Lorna, a friend of mine, recalls that in her last trip from Miami to San José, two of these seniors sat next to her, she being squeezed in the middle seat. The guy in the window seat was the closest replica of Woody Allen: short, thin, with big eye–glasses. The neighbor in the aisle seat was just the opposite: big, fat and with hair as white as sugar. Both are drinking Scotch and are in a talkative mood. Lorna who is also interested in the subject of sex tourism, initiates the conversation with Woody Allen's replica:

- "Is this your first time in Costa Rica?"
- "Not at all –he responds– It is my fourth time." Lorna asks the same question to her other neighbor
- "This is my twelfth visit"- he answers with a sardonic smile. The man already smells like alcohol.
- "Where are you headed in Costa Rica?" Insists Lorna.
- "I am headed to San José"- answers the fat man. The other guy nods in agreement.
- "So you are not on holidays?" Continues Lorna, who knows that if you are headed to the city; it is unlikely that you'd be on vacation.
- "No, no –replies our Woody Allen. We are on vacation and on adventures, but our target is Hotel Del Buey."

No more information is necessary. In the same way gay people used to reveal their sexual orientation by indicating they would visit Deja Vu Bar in San José, sex tourists only need to mention Hotel Del Buey and everyone knows what they are talking about. This hotel is the largest sex tourist establishment in the region, a place only rivaled by Campo Alegre in Curazao.

Several articles in the press and in academia have compared Costa Rica's sexual tourism boom with the one that made Thailand a sexual paradise for foreign tourists in the 1980s. Mariela Jimenez writes in the Associated Press "Costa Rica struggles with growing reputation as sex tourism Mecca."[1] In another article for the same agency she adds: "Tourism in general has become Costa Rica's most profitable industry over the 90's, thanks to its pristine beaches and spectacular volcanoes, as well as its reputation as a peaceful oasis in an unsettled region. And with Southeastern Asian countries like Thailand and the Philippines cracking down on sex tourism, Central America is emerging as a new hot spot for the sex trade, children's advocates say."[2]

In Costa Rica, according to IPS, adult prostitution is an unregulated, growing industry that is currently exploiting women from Central America, the Caribbean and Europe. In an article entitled: *Innocence for Sale: A Quarter of*

Costa Rica's Sex–tourists comes from the US,[3] the author wrote that "many of Costa Rica's children are being forced into prostitution by poverty and abuse, and the booming sex tourism industry is only too happy to put them to work." Bruce Harris, director of Casa Alianza (Covenant House) told IPS that "This is a growing business, and every day we hear more reports" of women caught up in the trade.[4] Costa Rica, like Thailand, has become a Mecca for sexual tourism.[5] Harris believes the invasion is led by 60–year–olds from the North who travel in search of young women and men. Jeremy Seabrook in the preface to the second edition of his book, *Travel in the Skin Trade. Tourism and the Sex Industry*, includes Costa Rica as a sexual tourist's Mecca.[6]

In 1989, tourism became the main source of income in Thailand, something similar to what happened in Costa Rica in 1992. Official estimates say that there are 85,000 sex workers in Thailand, 32% of them in Bangkok. The Thai Red Cross Society considers that the number can range between 200,000 and 800,000 sex workers. According to official data, Thailand has approximately 5,800 establishments that provide sexual services, 43% are brothels, 5.5% are bars/night–clubs and 3.8% are massage parlors. The remaining thirty eight percent are among the category of "others."[7] In addition, it is estimated that there are 650,000 people infected with AIDS or 1% of the population. In the north, where most sex workers come from, 7% of the population has become infected with the virus.[8]

As we will see, sexual tourism in Costa Rica has experienced a boom of its own. The "mongers" themselves recognize the rising trend despite their attempts to keep it affordable and small. The administrator of CostaRicaTicas.com recognizes that "The more the ex patriot population grows from guys from the US and Canada, the more the word gets out. I have also found that during the 'dry' season, or high season, the more mongers frequent 'our paradise'. The hotels are always booked up full from January thru March." Romulus, another sexual tourist, is unhappy with this boom. According to him, "It really bothers me to see so many american's (sic) down there now. It has rapidly become a mongers' paradise which will result in bitchy attitudes from the women and probably mechanical sex who will demand $100 who will not budge."[9]

According to figures supplied by official sources at international airports, 556,412 tourists visited Costa Rica from January through May of 2005, an increase of 23.5% over the same period last year. The records at Juan Santamaría and Daniel Oduber (Liberia) airports show the arrival of 450,478 tourists the first three months in 2005.[10] The data does not include the arrival of tourists on cruise ships or overland, therefore the actual number of visitors is higher. The majority of these tourists come to Costa Rica on holiday. (Table 3)

For the year 2002, there were a total of 1,113,360 tourists that came to Costa

Rica. Of these, 422,222 came from the United States. [11] In 2004, an estimated 1,5 million tourists visited Costa Rica, and in 2005, the figure rose to 1,9 million, mainly from the United States and Europe. From Miami, flight time is two hours and twenty minutes; the ticket costs around three hundred dollars, one third of the price of a Miami–Rio ticket. Astroglide, a monger, indicates the reason of his choosing Costa Rica over some other destinations. "I can get to CR for $313 right now. I can go to work . . . work almost a full day . . . catch a non–stop after work and be banging a chica in the Del Buey by 10 pm that Night! [12]

In 2005, La Nación, the main Costa Rican newspaper, recorded a 25% rise in tourism compared to the previous year. Another report in the same journal stated that the Juan Santamaría airport was ready to collapse due to the 2.7 million passengers. [13] The main reasons American tourists travel to Costa Rica are pleasure and recreation. (Table 2)

This boom has not gone unnoticed by Covenant House (Casa Alianza), an NGO that fights children's sexual exploitation. The organization claims there are 40 websites dedicated to promote sexual tourism to Costa Rica. [14] Bruce Harris, Executive Director, reports that thousands of Americans and Europeans are using Costa Rica as a sexual escapade. [15] His organization has fought to put these "sexual exploiters" into prison. Ironically, Harris was recently caught in the sex trade business. According to Reuters, "Covenant House has dismissed Mr. Harris because he recently paid a 19–year–old Honduran boy for sexual favors in a Tegucigalpa motel." Harris had admitted to "behaving in an incorrect manner."[16]

Sex tourists themselves recognize that Costa Rica is changing. Dallasman writes a history of the sex trade in *CostaRicaTicas.com*, a sex forum on Costa Rica. He believes that too much propaganda will deteriorate the place.

> *Up to a few years ago, the trade was much smaller, and the vast majority of the ladies that were working were semi–pros, i.e.: housewives, teachers, legal secretaries, etc. working a night or two a month to augment their income.*
> *I really liked it much more when that was the rule, not the exception. The scourge of Crack cocaine, as well as 'speed' in its many forms have also found its way along with some of these ladies, and all of the unwanted baggage that comes with this has also made its way to Costa Rica.*
>
> *As far as the ladies, several things happened a few years ago. A massive influx of non Tica ladies, mainly from Colombia, Nicaragua, the Dominican Republic, as well as some Eastern European countries changed the face of the hobby. The good is increased numbers, selection, and quality. The bad is now about 80–90% of the ladies are true 'pros'. Nothing wrong with that, but the GFE (girlfriend relationship) factor goes way down. You can still find the semi–pro's, but it is becoming harder, and harder to do.*

My personal opinion is shhhhhhhhhhhh, don't tell anyone else about this place, it is already spoiled my too many Ugly Americans.[17]

Sexual services are promoted by hotels, travel agencies, and escort services and even by fishing trip promoters. Sex workers can be delivered to the client's hotel door in Guanacaste. Clients can order a woman for an entire trip or one for every night at beach hotels. "Didn't you like what was brought to you?" "*No hay problema*" says the information in one brochure. "You can exchange her at no extra cost."

An American tourist in Guanacaste tells us the story of how one can be serviced "professionally." The company he hired brought to his room a sex worker he "did not have good chemistry with." He called right away the office and complained, "The woman was not as hot as I expected." "Did you have sex with her?"- The receptionist inquired. "I only kissed her once"- he responded. "As long as no penetration or oral sex has been performed"- the woman informed him– "You can return her without any charge." Three hours later, the company sent him another sex worker. "Irma, was a lovely whore –says this monger– and we hit it right along. We went dancing and partying all night and she was "*muy caliente*" and had "wonderful tits." The man was so happy that he would recommend this company to all his friends. "If you can return a damaged item" –he indicates with humor– "You will be a satisfied customer." [18]

Men and women, old and young, heterosexual and homosexual, participate in the new sex trade. In places like Quepos, sex workers specialize in young American men who are too shy to approach local girls. Costa Rican gigolos do their part with young American women who want to try something different in the tropics. [19] "*Ticas* are happy when the tourists leave because they can get their men back," a taxi driver in Quepos stated.

Despite the sex tourist boom, the comparison with Thailand is not yet deserved. In that country, 70% of the tourists go there only for sex, whereas in Costa Rica it might be between 5% and 10%. The number of Costa Rican establishments that cater to the sex industry is no more than fifty.

American tourists do not limit themselves to Costa Rica. There is a growing community of "mongers" that travel to and from other Latin American and Southeast Asian countries. They report to each other about the places, the expenses, the women, and everything there is to know about each site. Rio de Janeiro, Brazil, for example, is quite popular among mongers who frequent Costa Rica. They report that the women and the prices in Rio are better than in San José. Nevertheless, they also indicate that Rio is more commercial than Costa Rica and that the GFE (friendship relationship with the woman) experience is better in this Central American nation. Others are traveling to Granada in Nicaragua. There is now a direct flight from Liberia to Granada that makes it more affordable. American tourists list the nightclubs in this Central American city and report to have found a greater number of sex workers for much lower prices. Panama is becoming another option. Some mongers find this nation more modernized than Costa Rica and recommend it as the next stop for those who want something different. Finally, many of the tourists who go to San José also travel to Bogota, Colombia. After all, many of the sex workers in Costa Rica and in Panama are "*colombianas*" and many clients want to have the "real" experience in the women's native land. They also say that sex workers are cheaper in this South American nation than in San José. Thailand is the most popular site for American mongers and 40% of those sampled at www.costaricaticas.com find it their favorite destination. 18% prefer Brazil and other Latin countries; 9% rather go to Asian destinations, and 13% like East European destinations better.[20]

Given Costa Rica's attraction to American tourists, whichever place becomes the next sex Mecca in the region, it is doubtful that it will totally displace this Central American nation. On the contrary, whatever sexual "Monger culture" is being developed, it is more likely that it will be exported to other Central American nations. Joe1015 gives us his reasons:

These are my reasons that make my heart and soul feel so good about costa rica.

In San José, whenever I look towards the horizon I can see the beautiful mountains. I appreciate looking at mountains because Florida is as flat as a pancake and has boring terrain.
I like the cool breezes in san josé. It is a short and cheap flight from Florida.

Whenever I look at the women, they look back with an innocent smile. In the states the women look back with an attitude of "what the phuck are you looking at pervert ?

Costa Rica is a third world country and some parts of it are dirty and unkept, but this is what gives it character and charm.

I like the fact that most of the locals are 'happy go lucky' and friendly.

When I am physically in costa rica, I am there to relax, de–stress and play with beautiful sweet chicas. I am on vacation and for a brief moment I no longer think about work and other daily responsibilities back in the states.

On my first trip I was overly cautious and worried about my safety. After my third trip I feel very comfortable walking around San José.

Some of the crt guys I have met have made my trips much more enjoyable.

One of the main reasons I like costa rica is that the 'renting' of chicas is legal. I can have any girl I want there.

The fruits, pineapple and coffee taste better there.

Costa Rica is therapy for my mental health and emotions. [21]

Notes

1. AP, Sunday, November 28, 1999
2. http://www.friends–partners.org/partners/stop–traffic/1999/0565.html
3. Mother Jones.com News, 10 October, 2000
4. http://www.friends–partners.org/partners/stop–traffic/1999/1442.html
5. Jeremy Seabrook, *Travel in the Skin Trade: Tourism and the Sex Industry.* London: Pluto Press 2001.
6. Ibid, p. 10.
7. Hnin Hnin Pyne, *Aids and Prostitution in Thailand: A Study of Burmese Prostitutes in Ranong,* Master Thesis, (Massachusetts Institute of Technology, May 1992, p.21.
8. Chris Ryan and Michael Hall, *Sex Tourism and Liminalities,* Routledge, New York– London, 2001, p.48.
9. http://www.costaricaticas.com/phpbb2/viewtopic.php?t=1427
10. Tico Times, Feb 27, 2004
11. Costa Rican Tourist Board, http://www.costarica.com/Home/Business/Costa_Rica_in_Facts,_Numbers,_%7Damp;_Statistics/Tourism_%7Damp;_Visitor_Information/Tourism_Statistics
12. http://www.costaricaticas.com/phpBB2/viewtopic.php?t=4663
13. La Nación, San José, Costa Rica, September 1, 2004, p.15A.
14. Casa Alianza, *Regional Investigation on Trafficking, Prostitution, Child Pornography and Sex Tourism with Children in Central America and Mexico,* info@ casa–alianza.org, 2001.
15. Ibid, p. 10.
16. Periódico La Nación, September 17, 2004, p. 1.
17. http://www.costaricaticas.com/phpbb2/viewtopic.php?t=3182
18. http://www.costaricaticas.com/phpbb2/viewtopic.php?t=3182
19. Ronnie Shaw, *Fantasy Voyages: Exploration of White Male's Participation in the Sex Industry,* The Berkely McNair Research Journal (81)
20. http://www.costaricaticas.com/phpbb2/viewtopic.php?t=1759
21. http://www.costaricaticas.com/phpbb2/viewtopic.php?t=2821

2. Sex or going fishing?

Jeff, who looks like Woody Allen, is the guy sitting next to Lorna on the American Airlines flight to Costa Rica. He tells her while eating pretzels –a sign that flight service has been reduced to the bare minimum in recent years– that he first came to Costa Rica only to lay at the beach. He decided to spend some time in Flamingo, a beautiful spot on the Pacific where Elizabeth Taylor used to own a property. Back then, he was still married and was traveling with his wife. After Flamingo, they decided to visit another tourist spot in Jaco Beach.

His wife spent all day under the sun and decided to take a long nap in the afternoon. "Honey, go and take a walk through the town, I am so burned that I can hardly move," she recommended to him. Jeff decided to do as told and strolled along through the narrow streets filled with tourists and locals. As he passed Jaco's restaurants, he noticed two beautiful and friendly women who winked at him. The man winked back and gave them his best and friendliest smile. They returned the gesture and invited him to sit down with them. The women spoke good English and after some chit–chat, invited him to meet them later that evening at Bar Whole Wood –an American hang–out. Jeff hesitated at first since he knew his wife would not be interested in visiting a nightclub. Nevertheless, once he returned to the hotel, he found his wife sleeping like a log and decided not to wake her. "Honey, if you wake up, don't worry about me I will be watching TV in the lobby."- He wroteher in a note.

Anita and María, Jeff's acquaintances, were sitting at the bar all dressed up and looking, according to him, amazing. They had now heavy make–up, tight *manganos* and see–through blouses. Jeff could not refrain from complimenting them by telling them they looked *"muy calientes."* Suddenly, Anita asked him to slow dance with her and Jeff accepted her invitation. Dancing turned him on so much that five minutes later –and $75 less in his pocket– he was getting oral sex under the table. He paid $75 more and had sex with María in the men's toilet.

"Am I being too frank with you?" Jeff asked Lorna. He had no problem in being quite open to a woman he hardly knew and that he probably would never see again. Sex tourists like to talk and brag about their sexual lives, be it with men and/or women and.

"Not at all" –responded Lorna. "Please continue…

"There is not that much to add." He said. "This incident opened my eyes and appetites to new experiences. I decided that the next time I'd come to Costa Rica, my wife should stay in Wisconsin. The woman cannot stand so much sun," he said mischievously.

Some experts believe that Jeff's transition from eco to sex tourism is quite common. Ryan et al. opine that eco tourists want to enliven their senses through by being with what could be considered "wild" and "primitive" nature. The whole body becomes involved in the pursuit of pleasure and the step from being massaged by the warm waters of the Pacific to having the sensuous mouth of a local caressing one's genitals, is a very short one.

> *Sun bathing brings not only the possibility of a suntan, but also the sense of sun upon the skin, warmth and a pleasure. From sensuality to sexuality is a stepped procedure. And from sexuality to intercourse is but a farther graduation based upon payment.* [1]

The number of tourists who engage in sex tourism, then, can be greater if we add up those who come on holidays to Costa Rica and also engage in sex tourism by accident or as a sideline activity. O' Connel et al. also found this pattern in their study on sex tourism in the Caribbean.

> *Moreover, men who would not necessarily practice prostitution at home are able to do so while on holiday abroad due to the preconceptions that what occurs in Third World countries is "not really prostitution" and that the "girls" are "not really like prostitutes."* [2]

One clear example of such ambiguity was the group known as the "Michigan Boys" who came to Costa Rica to go "fishing." They were "eco–tourists" but as Ryan and Hall write, eco tourism and sex tourism have more in common than usually thought.

The Michigan Boys came to Costa Rica in a Charter on May 16, 2004. The group included the rich and famous of Detroit's society. The men were leaders of this city's business and political elites; others were members of the US Government; some professional football players also came along. There were 167 of them, the type of men who should not have any problem in picking women back home. They told their wives and lovers that they were embarking in a fishing trip to the Pacific. They had in their hands the most state–of– the art equipment to prove it. They got together, reads the newspaper article, "before dawn at the Macomb County restaurant where bartender Angelo Nucci has served up this annual junket for nine years now." The articles continues: "But about six hours later, when they arrived at a small Costa Rican airfield, the men stepped down into a faraway land where they suspected no one would be watching or care how they were greeted by natives who couldn't have been friendlier if they'd been paid."

"So what could be wrong with this picture? ..." asks the journalist. The answer forecasts a tropical storm:

The fishing expedition was not actually interested in catching fish: "Apparently many of the beautiful Costa Rican women were paid –and for much more than that friendly welcome they gave the Michigan Boys at the airport. When the Boys' buses arrived at their luxury seaside hotel, and for the duration of their five–day stay, dozens of prostitutes were waiting to party. One hotel worker put it simply to our hidden camera: "The men and women are up to 5 A.M. partying. The girls go from guy to guy."[3]

This was no isolated phenomenon. Many of ecotourism and fishing packages end up the same way. A famous Website, for example, offers more "fishing" tours to Costa Rica and the baits provided are not necessarily worms:

> *Just another option . . . I am marketing for a new tour biz here in CR called "Gone Fishin Costa Rica Tours." While they have had issues getting their website up . . . they do have over 24 girlfriends waiting to hook up for traveling with Gringos . . . The GOne Fishin biz includes security, translation services and a welcome party to meet the girls before you are committed, and great combination hotel and transport packages besides . . . .*[4]

Sex tourism does not only involve sex with prostitutes. Many of the tourists also come to have sex with what they call "non–pro" Costa Rican women.

There is significant evidence that suggest that many tourists, both female and male, are not adverse to sexual adventure if it happens during a holiday. Clark and Clift found within their sample of British tourists in Malta that 7,7% admitted to having a "romantic relationship" while on holiday. Gillies and Slack, in a sample of 541 holidaymakers, found that 5% had had sexual relationships with people other than their normal partner while on holiday.[5]

Mongers also share their experiences with others about the large possibilities in engaging in sex with Costa Rican women who do not work in prostitution. Administrator 3 admitted, contrary to popular belief, that it is much easier to have sex with women who do not work in prostitution on the first date.

The American tourist, he thinks, does not need to put too much energy in seducing them as women seem willing to be approached. Dman suggests American men should go out around 11 am and "dress up in nice slacks and shirt, and head down to la avenida central near the banks around the green space." According to him, one has to wait for local women who work at banks and Government buildings to go out for lunch and then "watch and wait. It is all about eye contact. If they return your look and smile with their eyes, then approach them." This monger recognized having "scored dozens of women" in this manner. "They are all eager to have dinner and I would say that more times than not, after dinner we end going out for drinks and end up at their place." These women –he believes– are "hornier" than their American counterparts as "First date is way different than with gringas." [6]

These sexual encounters are not uncommon as a survey from www.costaricaticas.com shows 25% of the men in this sample had sex with more than three "non–pro" Costa Rican women. 11% has had intercourse with more than six women.

This is an interesting phenomenon, as mongers do not seem to have major problems in Costa Rica to have sex without having to pay for it. Nevertheless, they also confess that what attract them to sex workers is that there are no–strings attached.

Sex workers who cater to tourists

We found 543 sex workers and 219 American tourists in 15 different sex establishments during our mapping of September 4, 2004 (slow tourist season in Costa Rica). We did not visit 20 other places listed in the sex tour guides. According to our informants, these smaller establishments have an average of 15 sex workers, which means another 300 sex workers in our tally. The total of sex workers, therefore, in a low season night could be around 800.

It is very difficult, from this data, to estimate the total number of sex workers that cater to tourists. In certain places, such as Hotel Del Buey, the turnover is very high. It is estimated by some informants that less than 20% of the women are "regulars." Some of them come once a month and others once a year. "If I can't make enough at my beauty parlor," says Mariana, "I come here to make some extra bucks. I come to Del Buey only when I need cash." If we speculate that, in a given night, between 800 and 1,000 prostitutes work at the sex tourism establishments and that this number could be roughly a 10% of the total, according to our informants, the number of sex workers could range from 8,000 to 10,000.

Hotel	American tourists	Sex workers
Hotel Del Buey	110	240
Tea Amargo	95	115

Visit to Night Clubs
Dates: September 4, 8 and 11, 2004

Night Club	Costa Rican males	American tourists	Sex workers
Bar 1	4	2	20
Bar 2	6	0	18
Bar 3	8	5	23
Bar 4	4	5	15
Bar 5	125	0	12
Bar 6	84	2	20
Bar 7	6	0	15

Visit to Massage Parlors
September 11, 2004

Massage Parlor	Costa Rican males	American tourists	Sex workers	Price of sexual act
MP 1	12	8	25	$40
MP 2	1	0	4	$30
MP 3	3	0	4	$22
MP 4	0	2	7	$55
MP 5	2	0	10	$45
MP 6	4	0	15	$22

Sex tourists

According to Michael B. Farrell, 80% of sex tourists in Costa Rica are American. [7] Since tourists usually stay at a hotel and some of these hotels are exclusively for sex tourism, it is much easier to calculate the client's numbers. The hotels that allow tourists to take women into their rooms are dedicated to the sex trade. Families and business people do not frequent these places.

Nevertheless, we should not assume that prostitutes are absent in American chain hotels. Chaser writes that he was able to get two sex workers at San José's

Charriot: "I stay about a half hour away from San José at the Charriot Costa Rica. So you can probably add an hour on for their time. I was there last January and I played $300 to a VERY Beautiful young lady who was my true companion from about 10pm until about 3 or 4 am. I was sure she was a bargain."[8] Nucknuts confirmed that the Charriott has a good variety of sex workers working in its premises, but the higher quality of the hotel drives prices up. Chaser complained that the Charriot "is charging too much for the women." "The girls do expect more if you are at the Charriott. Not only due to the time but they know you have to be 'high–end' to stay there."[9] Tman, on the other hand, has the opinion that the Charriot also has sex workers with prices no higher than at Del Buey: "I know guys that stay at the Charriot and never pay more than $100 . . . for all night sometimes . . . not that I understand wanting a prostitute ALL NIGHT."[10] Gringotim thinks that the Charriott might be further away from "the Gulch"[11], or the prostitution area where Del Buey is, but this does not entitle the place to be more expensive. Chaser believes that being further away from the Gulch "doesn't justify *mucho dinero*."[12]

Hotel Del Buey, Hotel El Duende and others nearby are part of downtown San José's "Gulch," area. These are establishments that cater only to sex tourists. Given this fact, we can provide a rough estimate of the number of clients in the red–light district based on their occupancy rate and the number of rooms. Needless to say, as we have seen above, not all sex tourists stay at these hotels. Some also rent apartments in downtown or stay with friends or relatives.

Hotel	Number of rooms	Occupancy
Hotel 1	200	50%
Hotel 2	87	50%–60%
Hotel 3	96	100%
Hotel 4	116	100%
Hotel 5	110	50%–60%
Hotel 6	74	60%
Hotel 7	30	100%
Hotel 8	40	50%
Hotel 9	69	50%
Hotel 10	104	100%
Total	926	

According to these data:

1. The average occupancy rate for these hotels is 72%. In a regular day, there are 667 occupied rooms, of which two men occupy half of them. This gives

us approximately 1000 persons per day. If the average stay in Costa Rica is seven days, there will be 4,000 men per month and 48,000 men per year.

2. According to our ethnographic observations and data from the sex forums, many American sex tourists stay either at Hotel Del Buey or at Hotel El Duende. Both hotels have a total of 200 rooms and are usually 100% full. The waiting period for a room is of a month and a half. In a given month these two hotels will have approximately 1,200 men (average of seven days per person and half of the rooms).
3. Since there are many more hotels that cater to sex tourists and that not all sex tourists go to these hotels, the minimum could be around 20,000 men and the maximum around 50,000 men; that is, between 5% to 10% of the total number of American visitors. The administrators of Costa Rica's sex forums indicate that only 5% to 10% of mongers know about the websites. CostaRicaticas.com has 2,500 subscribers and many more thousands as guests. If the relationship established by its administrators between loggers versus actual mongers is correct (5–10% of mongers are members of the Websites), a total of 30,000 to 50,000 "mongers" is not a far–fetched figure. If we add up to this group, those American and Canadian ex patriots who live in Costa Rica and who also participate in the sex trade, the numbers could double. Davidson, one of the most knowledgeable experts on the subject of sex tourism, cites a 1994 study estimating that more than 30,000 Americans and several thousand more Canadians had retired to Costa Rica. Many of the single men among them were described as "sex–pats," ex patriates who retired there not just for the climate, tax breaks, and other advantages but also for the "easy and cheap sexual access to their preferred sexual objects."[13] If we include the "sex pats," the total number of sex tourists might be between 50,000 and 80,000.

One of the interesting facts of Costa Rica's sexual tourism is the concentration of a large number of the American tourists in a few hotels. These hotels have not followed a thought out plan of development but have rather benefited from urban decay and loss of customers by former tourist hotels in downtown San José. This was the case of Barrio Amón, a very classy neighborhood in San José that started to sell its run–down buildings some decades ago. Hotel Del Buey, for example, was bought in this area before the tourist boom in Costa Rica for approximately one million dollars, and now it is being estimated to be worth more than 15 million dollars. The same can be said about Hotel El Duende. This was a proper hotel for business executives some years ago; nevertheless, it became too noisy and polluted before it became a place for picking up sex workers. These two hotels get around of 75% of the sex tourists who are members of CostaRica.Ticas.com. The rest goes to other hotels nearby, such as Hotel 2 or Hotel 3 in downtown San José, or other "no mongers hotels."[14]

Hotel Del Buey is the favorite place for sex among sex tourists, as the poll in Costaricaticas.com shows. The members are asked where "would you like to go if you only had one more sexual opportunity in your live." 65% answers that they would go to Hotel Del Buey. 30% say they rather spend it at MP's such as MP5, MP 1 and MP 2. 4% indicate they would spend this last sexual experience at Tea Amargo, a nightclub owned by the same company that runs Hotel Del Buey. Not one single member suggests that he would spend his last sexual act with his wife or with his partner back home. [15]

On a single night in September 2004, we found 250 sex workers at Hotel Del Buey and 95 at Tea Amargo. These two places concentrate 75% of the American clientele and the same company owns both. This is rather unique and very different from other sexual Mecca such as Rio or Thailand. During high season in January, there were 700 sex workers at Hotel Del Buey and 500 sex tourists.

"Mongers" or sexual tourists spend their days having sex in such hotels without having to step out of them. They resemble the gay baths of the 1980's in the United States. A monger usually has sex three or more times a day, with more than one woman. Dcr37 reports having had sex with 37 sex workers in 10 days:

> *no it was not my 37th trip, it was my 3rd. but what i did was have 37 chicks in a ten day period.....yes it was heaven. i wish i could remember all the names, and will try to figure it out, with the help of my videos [sic] and pics* [16]

The large concentration of mongers and sex workers in a few hotels must be taken into account as part of the Costa Rican excitement. One walks into Hotel Del Buey and is struck by the number of both sex workers and clients. It adds a sort of legitimacy to an activity that is liminal. It brings men together in spaces where sex can be openly recognized and discussed, something many admit having problems doing back home. It creates a culture that not only shares its liking for paid sex but also its life philosophy. Carlos, a dealer, thinks that Del Buey is a sort of big Roman–type orgy room. It mesmerizes men and helps them jump into a holiday from daily life. He has seen American tourists who come to see the place, with no intentions of engaging in sex, get caught immediately into this culture and remain hooked to it. "You get in here, feeling like any other sixty–year old man, not that attractive and not so competitive any more in the game of romance, and see hundreds of beautiful women trying to get your attention, willing to please you and to have sex with you and then you feel like a young man again and you do not want to lose this feeling anymore, something that will happen when you walk out of Del Buey's front door. You come back and you come back because you no longer want to leave for good." Lucy, a sex worker, believes it is not only paid sex that turns this industry into such an addictive drug; "Prostitutes don't care about good looks. You have a large number of women who are not turned on by youth. This is what makes these places so enticing."

Notes

1. Chris Ryan and C. Michael Hall, *Sex Tourism. Marginal people and liminalities,* London: Routledge, 2001, p.7.

2. O'Connell Davidson and Sanchez Taylor, "Fantasy Islands: Exploring the Demand for Sex Tourism." In *Sun, Sex, and Gold: Tourism and Sex Work in the Caribbean,* edited by Kamala Kempadoo, 37–54.Lanham: Rowman and Littlefield, 1999, p.43

3. http://www.wxyz.com/wxyz/ys_investigations/article/0%2C2132%2CWXYZ_15949_2892599%2C00.html

4. http://costaricasex.board.dk3.com/viewtopic.php?topic=626&forum=1&22

5. In Chris Ryan and C. Michael Hall, *Sex Tourism. Marginal people and liminalities,* London: Routledge, 2001, p.60

6. http://costaricasex.board.dk3.com/viewtopic.php?topic=626&forum=1&22

7. Michael B. Farrell, "Global campaign to police sex tourism," Christian Science Monitor (Article on–line); available at http://csmweb2.emcweb.com/2004/0422/p11s01wogl.htm; accessed June 30,2004.

8. http://www.costaricaticas.com/phpBB2/viewtopic.php?t=4442

9. http://www.costaricaticas.com/phpBB2/viewtopic.php?t=4442

10. http://www.costaricaticas.com/phpBB2/viewtopic.php?t=4442

11. The name is used since the Hotel Del Buey is downhill in San José and sex tourists must "climb up" to the other sex spots.

12. http://www.costaricaticas.com/phpBB2/viewtopic.php?t=4442

13. http://www.fas.harvard.edu/~drclas/publications/revista/Tourism/hannum.html

14. http://www.costaricaticas.com/phpbb2/viewtopic.php?t=1227&highlight=poll

15. http://www.costaricaticas.com/phpBB2/viewtopic.php?t=4361

16. http://costaricasex.board.dk3.com/viewtopic.php?topic=716&forum=1&22

3. Origins and characteristics

Sex tourism is tourism, partially or fully for the purpose of having sex, often with prostitutes. One term for a sex tourist is "sexpat." When travel opportunities opened up to a growing segment of the middle class in the mid–19th century, including that of the United States, sex tourism evolved into a common activity. As many European countries became wealthier, clients expanded their search for sex into other regions, such as the Caribbean and northern Africa, where prices for sex were more moderate. [1]

Wealthy people have always traveled to distant parts of the world to see great buildings or other works of art; to learn new languages; or to taste new cuisine. As long ago as the time of the Roman Republic places such as Baiae were popular coastal resorts for the rich. The terms tourist and tourism were first used as official terms in 1937 by the League of Nations. Tourism was defined as "people traveling abroad for periods of over twenty four hours." [2]

Mass travel could not really begin to develop until two things occurred.

a) Improvements in communications allowed the transport of large numbers of people in a short space of time to places of leisure interest, and
b) Greater numbers of people began to enjoy thc benefits of leisure time. A major development was the invention of the railways, which brought many of Britain's seaside towns within easy distance of Britain's urban centers.

The father of modern mass tourism was Thomas Cook who, on 5 July 1841, organized the first package tour in history, by chartering a train to take a group of temperance campaigners from Leicester to a rally in Loughborough, some twenty miles away. Cook immediately saw the potential for business development in the sector, and became the world's first tour operator. [3]

Some argue that sex tourism started in the Americas with the arrival of

Christopher Columbus and the exchange of trinkets for sex with the indigenous women. Ann Barger Hannum says, "Considerable research supports the theory that, along with potatoes, tobacco, and other commodities, Columbus and his crew also brought the first cases of syphilis to the New World."[4] Eduard Said writes that in the New West Indies the phenomenon of sexual exploitation of Colonial peoples is rather old and that "Western men have long projected racist fantasies onto the 'primitive'/natural Other."[5]

These authors suggest possible reasons for seeking sex in another country or region:

- More relaxed morality laws (for some people a lower age of consent may also be relevant)
- Less rigorous enforcement of laws
- Cheaper rates (typically due to traveling from a economically wealthy country to a poorer one)
- More anonymity / privacy
- Finding certain ethnic groups more attractive
- Preferring the "work ethics" of foreign prostitutes to those of one's own country
- Finding sex in tropical surroundings and a hot climate more arousing

Common destinations for sex tourists include Brazil, Thailand, Cambodia, Costa Rica, and Cuba. Since the collapse of the Iron Curtain, Russia, Hungary and the Czech Republic have also become popular destinations for sex tourists. In many of those destinations, sex tourism is still only a small percentage of overall prostitution, with most prostitutes serving local men.

Destinations for female sex tourism include the Caribbean, Costa Rica, Gambia, and some North African countries. This variant of sex tourism usually doesn't include outright prostitution, as some local males consider it a kind of sport to pick up female tourists, since sex with local women out of a committed relationship is hard to get for them.

While most sex tourists only engage in this activity with other adults, a small percentage actively look for adolescent or even younger prostitutes, while others are not very selective either way, regarding age. Several countries, such as Costa Rica, have severe laws against having sex with children.

According to Ronnie Shaw, Thailand serves as a model illustrating the socio–economic, political, and cultural context that acts as a catalyst for the sex tourism trade. According to her, thousands of rural women were taken to the cities to satisfy a growing demand by American troops first, and of sexual tourists later. Shaw thinks, "Sheer economic need combined with American male patronage created a prostitution economy."[6]

She believes that in Costa Rica the same conditions were there for the sex industry to flourish. First of all, the country has undergone a similar process: "This mirrors Costa Rica where many women and children, uprooted due to cuts in social programs, provide personal services to western tourists."[7]

It might be politically correct to blame urbanization, rural uprootness and globalization for the increase of prostitution in Costa Rica. Nevertheless, this country does not seem to fit Shaw's model. There might be some connections between prostitution and globalization, but not those envisioned by her. First of all, the country was not undergoing a process of urbanization in the 1990's when the sex tourist industry took off (This had taken place after the 1960's). Secondly, there had never been American bases in her territory. Moreover, the country has no army and military bases. Finally, the country has had a massive immigration of Nicaraguan workers that reflects low unemployment.

There is poverty nonetheless, but the society is more egalitarian than most Latin American or Southeast Asian nations. Most sex workers who target the American sex tourist's demand are not Costa Ricans and therefore, are not engaging in prostitution because of poverty. On the contrary, Colombian or Dominican sex workers must have good sources of income back home to be able to afford the trip to Costa Rica and to be able to pay people to take care of their children and relatives. The local women who do come to the hotels and nightclubs that cater to American tourists are middle class, most of them employed and with at least secondary education.

The country does belong to the Third World and as Shaw points out, to the realm of the "other" and the "exotic." The population is mostly white or mestizo (Indian and Spanish) and different from the Anglo–Saxon phenotype. This might lead Americans to perceive Costa Rican society as more "traditional", "uncivilized" and "close to Nature" than the States and allow them to act in ways they would not dare to act back home: "You're getting down and dirty [culturally tabooed sex] and you're loving it! Admit it! You can't do this at home." Hence, a shift in ethics may exist because of the foreign atmosphere." –writes a sex tourist.[8]

American tourists comprise the greatest bulk of sex tourists simply because Costa Rica is close to the States and the country has a lower standard of living. Geographical proximity is not the only factor; if this were the case, Haiti would be a major sex tourist Mecca in the region. American men prefer light–skinned Ticas. You hardly find black Costa Rican sex workers in the Gulch.

Self–definition

Michel Foucault in his book "*The History of Sexuality*" argued that many sexual practices develop in a context in which those who act on them do not become aware that they constitute a sexual culture.[9] Before modernity, for example, men had sexual practices with other men and women with other women, without both groups acquiring what we now call a sexual identity. They might have thought that they were engaging in "Sodomy", but would never have considered being "homosexual." The perception of belonging to a sexual minority took, according to Foucault, centuries to develop.

In the case of sexual tourists, there is a growing sense of identity, not that different from homosexuals. First of all, sex tourists have created a non–pejorative definition of their practice that excludes terms such as "sex tourist" or "sex depredator." For them, men who pay for sex are "whoremongers", a word that is shortened to "mongers."

The dictionary defines "monger" as "A person promoting something undesirable or discreditable." A whoremonger is a man who likes paid sex.

Mongers do not see anything wrong in their preferences for young women who sell sex. They are aware that most people do not approve of them. Prolijo, for example, thinks "We may not personally consider what we do to be undesirable or discreditable. However, I would bet that most of us would not advertise our hobby to the general public, most of whom do not share our views."[10]

Being a "monger" is not just a sexual practice anymore. Fr. Lus thinks that a monger's additional trait, besides the attraction toward paid sex, is his rejection of committed relationships.

> *I am a whore–monger. I do not apologize for that. I love women –plural, not singular. I love sex. I have been married. That is a fine thing for some people, perhaps even for all people some of the time. It worked for me for only a limited number of years and then was a) not fun b) not pleasurable c) demanding and finally by mutual agreement, it was over. I have dated and had a few long term (6 months or more) 'relationships' but, due to my unwillingness to make such a relationship permanent and/or my preference for independence and maintaining my 'own space', that didn't work out...*
> *So, my answer –years ago– was to go to places where I could find available and affordable sex and companionship. First, I enjoyed the company of the whores in places like Amsterdam, Munich, Saigon, and Bangkok when I was in the service. Years later, it seemed natural to head down to Tijuana where I have now been going for 25+ years. In recent years I've tried Hong Kong, Jamaica and most recently, Costa Rica. .*[11]

Mongers themselves like to initiate their friends into their culture. Similarly to gays who like to bring other men out of the closet, mongers like to out their friends. It is fairly common to read in the Internet stories of how men entice each other to get involved in prostitution. A typical case is of a man who is in a holiday with his wife and gives a call to an American friend who lives in Costa Rica. The monger invites him for a drink at the Blue Queen in Hotel Del Buey. After being introduced to the women and being told how to get them, the man decides to come back next time without his wife. "A new monger is born!" –He writes with pride.

Sex tourists are growing in numbers. Prostitution in the States, after the sexual revolution in the 1960's, seemed destined to decline as a middle–class activity, but it seems to be on the rise again among males who visit Third World countries. Many North Americans, according to Express321, "have come out of the closet" and "Packs of mongers show up every week. Even young guys are going in real numbers now, many of them can get young ass for free at home or for the price of a meal and a few drinks. But I am sure they like a sure thing with a hot chick." [12]

In our ethnographic observations we found many young and attractive American tourists in the nightclubs and massage parlors. Some of them are visiting relatives in Costa Rica, are in student–exchange programs or simply vacationing. Many public American figures participate in the sex trade. R. W., for example, a famous football player of the Miami Dolphins, was spotted at Hotel Del Buey. In Quepos, for example, there are sex workers who target exclusively young male and female Americans. American women may feel a sense of power hiring the services of a sex worker and thus break away from dating patterns in the United States. On the other hand, the men find it much easier to pay for sex than to approach local women. Cristina, who works in a hotel that caters to young Americans, asserts that these young tourists would never confess to their peers back home what they do in Quepos; "But they pay for sex like the older ones. They want sex in the tropics no matter the cost."

"Mongering" does not grow just in numbers but it is becoming incorporated into middle–class ceremonies, such as bachelor parties. Raffie, for example, is getting married. Nevertheless, he asks for help to older mongers as he is planning to have, along four of his friends, his bachelor party in Costa Rica.

> *Hi,*
> *My wedding party is going down for a final sendoff and I wonder if I can get some advice on arranging a wonderful time for 4 guys . . . 3 nights.*
> *We'd like to hang together . . . orgy–style . . . it's our first time to CR and we want it to be memorable.* [13]

He gets a good advice from RealmanK who thinks Raffie is heading for trouble. Once he gets into mongerland, the odds are that he will stay: "Don't go . . . you'll never go through with the wedding. Hell, you may never return home." [14]

Mongering might be coming age irrelevant, but not yet. Despite the participation of young mongers, the average sex tourist is still between 50–59 years of age (38%). A smaller group is between 40–49 years of age (27%). The rest is divided between the very young and the very old. Some sex tourists are in their eighties, and many more are between sixty and seventy years old. Marylin, a sex worker, tells us that the youngest man she has had is an American boy who was 13 years old. His uncle in a private party in Guanacaste introduced the kid to her. The oldest man she had been with was 92 years old. "He only wanted me to masturbate him and I learned he died three weeks later." [15]

Mongers live mainly in Florida, Midwest, Southwest, Northwest and the Mountain states. [16]

As of their physical appearance, 35% of those polled in CostaRicaTicas.com describe themselves as overweight, 31% thinks that they are "in shape", a similar percentage of mongers consider itself to be "average," and one percent thinks that it "can't see its shoes." [17]

One of the forum administrators who have met thousands of sexual tourists provides this humorous, but not far from the truth, description of the typical monger:

a. Middle aged single and only meets American women with tons of baggage and problems not to mention saggy tits and baggy asses.
b. Older guys that had given up getting any sort or sex.
c. Married guys that want and need variety and want to feel young and viral [sic] again, ie. looking for fountain of youth.
d. Single young guys frustrated with paying for expensive dates and getting no sex o very poor sex.
e. Guys that just like lots of sex and enjoy Latinas. [18]

Another sexual tourist, Don Giovani, explains that if they were all good–looking and young, most would not be mongering: "Of course, if we were all handsome young studs we wouldn't have to go to Costa Rica to have sex with beautiful young women." [19]

Monger's self–description fits how others see them. Lodge in his novel *Paradise News*, describes tourists dressed in shell suits and shorts– signs of being a tourist. "Both representations are concerned with a display for the body and nakedness or near nakedness are involved. Yet, the realism of the display is that it is not the appearance of glamorized bodies seen in pin–up calendars. The short, the fat, and the skinny are revealed and both tourists and prostitute have to come to the truth of their bodily appearance even while both hide and display the body at the same time."[20]

Sex tourists might generally be unattractive and old, but those not mean they can't find sex back home. On the contrary, many mongers report being sought by their American female counterparts and many do have sex with them. Nevertheless, when mongers talk about these sexual relationships, they claim to do it out of pity or pressure since they no longer feel attracted to wrinkles and saggy bodies. Happyman, for example, indicates that most mongers come to Costa Rica to get what is no longer attainable in the States, i.e. sex with beautiful women. It is their preference for youth that forces them to come to the Third World.

> *Vegas Bob planted a statement in my head that I can't get rid of. He said, in his big loud voice, "happyman, you will know you are not in CR when you go to the supermarket in the states and see a beautiful young girl behind the register..... that you just love and gives you a roaring hard on...........but, alas, you realize you can't have her. She is unattainable. That's when you'll know you are no longer in Costa Rica"*[21]

Finally, mongers enjoy sex and invest lots of energy into getting it. As a matter of fact, both groups have created establishments such as gay saunas or Hotel Del Buey to be able to have as much sex as possible. The sex forums are filled with posts of tourists who run from the airport to the massage parlors or to the hotel bars to pick up as many women as possible. There are cases of tourists who come to this country only for 24 hours and who end up having sex with more than 10 sex workers.

To buy sex, language is not a barrier. The majority of mongers do not speak Spanish. In the poll at CostaRicaTicas. com, only 4% of the sample knows how to speak Spanish.[22] The discussion forums are filled with questions concerning the meaning of words and advices on how to get by without speaking the language. The answers are usually that sex workers understand a little bit of English and that the only way they communicate with clients is by using Spanglish. Foreign sex workers that speak English, although only basic English, are the only exceptions.

In the interviews, sex workers also admitted the limiting aspect of Spanglish. Many of the sex workers stated that a lot of the communication is unclear and lends to many misunderstandings. In our ethnographic study, we found couples of North American men with sex workers who look, smile, kiss and touch each other and spend numerous minutes without speaking a word. Legman, for example, wants to know how to negotiate without words. He is concerned about not being able to understand anything but "it seems from your posts that although it may be a hindrance, it won't kill me!"[23] Sweet P., for example, did not know how to say in Spanish that he was ready to come. Unable to say this, he ejaculated in her mouth. He recognizes now that "It was hard when she didn't understand a thing I said. I guess I better work on my Spanish."[24] Lulu, a sex worker, believes that the major problem is not knowing what the client wants. She once asked for a condom in Spanish (preservativo) and the monger brought her a match (cerillo). Arlette wanted vaseline and Mike thought she wanted hair mousse. Christian wanted a Nicaraguan sex worker to perform oral sex and the woman thought he was asking for a mouthwash.

A tourist might find himself with a sex worker after years of having sex only with his wife. The woman doesn't understand his language. What does he do?

María thinks that many of her customers have missed the safe sex revolution because they were in monogamous relationships back in the United States. This is one of the reasons why they do not use condoms that much: they haven't met that many people with AIDS. In the poll taken at CostaRicaticas.com, most mongers admit not knowing straight people with AIDS.

I personally know at least one completely heterosexual person who has acquired HIV from heterosexual activity		
Yes	4%	[3]
No	95%	[61]
	Total Votes:	64 [25]

Some have not used a condom in years and others have never used one. "It is harder for them to learn to use condoms than for the younger generation"–she argues. Others have rekindled their sexual life thanks to the new sexual–enhancing drugs. These drugs allow them to have erections and penetrative sex after years of impotency. "Some customers don't like condoms because they are afraid of losing their hard–on" –Lupita confesses.

It is not difficult to anticipate that they will face serious communication problems with women who are usually half their age and from a different culture. Both the customer and the sex worker can easily fall into disagreements and disappointments over money, which increases the chances of violent and unsafe sex.

How do mongers negotiate with sex workers?

Romulus writes that there is no etiquette with regard to paying sex workers for their services. Some believe that it is better not to pay after the sexual act because "if you're horny as hell and she is hot, your ability to stand firm diminishes."[26] Sailor, on the other hand, sees payment as a small war. He argues that "he has beaten the shit out of two girls who insisted on being paid upfront." According to him, it is important not to give in because "you actually get some respect by standing your ground and having the session on your terms. I have seen it work in my favor numerous times. You can see in their eyes they understand you are a man who knows a woman's place in their culture."[27]

Joe1015 believes that sex workers should be paid first.[28] He thinks that in doing so he makes the women happy and less willing to trick him. Romulus, on the other hand, thinks that paying upfront is not a good idea: "The thing is I have stood my ground on a few occasions and it only led to pretty lame, mechanical sex." The reason is, he continues, that "women lose their incentives." He recognizes that once in the sexual act it is hard to negotiate the payment : "Guess I should have kicked her out but when your clothes are off and she is giving a BJ its a little difficult."[29] Finally, Express 321 thinks that the demand for money upfront is an American cultural influence in Costa Rica and recommends a compromise with it.[30]

Mongers do not know what to do about the money. In part it is recognition that the woman is having sex for material interest and this contradicts their fantasies. It also creates a burden for sex workers as they are forced to provide their service before getting paid for it. If for any reason their client is not satisfied with their services, he may feel entitled to reduce the agreed rate or as they themselves admit "kick the woman out." For this reason, sex workers feel more vulnerable to negotiate after the sexual act. Moreover, sex workers come from a culture that is less open about negotiating money and find it difficult to speak bluntly about the matter. Lucy states that she hates to be paid afterwards since the clients usually become less understanding after they have had their orgasm; "You feel them hostile after they come. They look for excuses not to pay." Gloria argues that her clients get upset when she stops her fellatio after several minutes. "They expect you to blow them for hours. Some don't have any juice left –after being having sex constantly– and they do not feel they need to come, ever…" This, according to her, is one of the greatest problems with the American clients.

American society is more homogenous than European and Latin American societies. In the United States there is a larger middle classs. A carpenter in the States can make as much money as a doctor or a lawyer in a Latin country. Since the cost of a 10–day sexual escapade for the American monger is approximately $2,200, this is an affordable expense to either the American working man or the middle class professional.

Despite the Costa Rican affordability, mongering seems to be more a middle class phenomenon. The sex forums are filled with posts from professional men with high incomes who seem highly educated and whose posts reveal psychological insights and awareness of international politics and culture. It is not the typical American working class guy who apparently comes to Costa Rica for sex.[31]

We found polls at the sex forums on the sex tourists' daily expenses. The majority indicated they spent less than $200 daily, excluding sex work. If this is added to the tally, the numbers increase to $300 a day.[32] The average total expense of the trip according to Xanadu, an expert from the sexual forum, is around $2200. This includes an average of 10 women at $90 each.[33]

If we calculate that the number of sexual tourists that visit Costa Rica per year is between 20,000 and 50,000, we can speculate that they can put in from $44 million to $110 million to the country's economy (this excludes the expats's expenses in Costa Rica). This is more than the country's exports of meat and sugar combined (Table 1). This data does not include money sent to sex workers to establish second houses, to purchase properties or to make investments in Costa Rica.

Notes

1. http://www.worldhistory.com/wiki/T/Tourism.htm
2. http://www.worldhistory.com/wiki/T/Tourism.htm
3. http://www.worldhistory.com/wiki/T/Tourism.htm
4. by Ann Barger Hannum,*Tricks of the Trade:Sex Tourism in Latin America* in: http://www.fas.harvard.edu/~drclas/publications/revista/Tourism/hannum.html
5. http://www.awigp.com/default.asp?numcat=sextour. Issue Number 5, March 2001.
6. Ronnie Shaw, *Fantasy Voyages: Exploration of White Male's Participation in the Sex Industry,* The Berkely McNair Research Journal (82).
7. Ronnie Shaw, *Fantasy Voyages: Exploration of White Male's Participation in the Sex Industry,* The Berkely McNair Research Journal (82)
8. Ronnie Shaw, *Fantasy Voyages: Exploration of White Male's Participation in the Sex Industry,* The Berkely McNair Research Journal (83)
9. Michell Foucault, *The History of Sexuality Vol. 1*, Vintage Books, 1990.
10. http://www.costaricaticas.com/phpbb2/viewtopic.php?t=82&postdays=0&postorder=asc&highlight
11. http://www.costaricaticas.com/phpbb2/viewtopic.php?t=97
12. http://www.costaricaticas.com/phpbb2/viewtopic.php?t=2856

13. http://216.157.152.197/phpbb2/viewtopic.php?t=3621
14. http://216.157.152.197/phpbb2/viewtopic.php?t=3621
15. http://www.costaricaticas.com/phpbb2/viewtopic.php?t=1643&highlight=poll
16. http://www.costaricaticas.com/phpbb2/viewtopic.php?t=1643&highlight=poll
17. http://www.costaricaticas.com/phpbb2/viewtopic.php?t=1725
18. http://www.costaricaticas.com/phpbb2/viewtopic.php?t=3401
19. Ibid.
20. Chris Ryan and Michael Hall, *Sex Tourism. Marginal People and Liminalities,* Routledge: London, 2001, p.4.
21. http://216.157.152.197/phpbb2/viewtopic.php?t=4031
22. http://www.costaricaticas.com/phpbb2/viewtopic.php?t=2623
23. http://www.costaricaticas.com/phpbb2/viewtopic.php?t=3126
24. http://www.costaricaticas.com/phpbb2/viewtopic.php?t=3126
25. http://www.costaricaticas.com/phpBB2/viewtopic.php?t=4954
26. http://www.costaricaticas.com/phpbb2/viewtopic.php?t=3122&highlight
27. http://www.costaricaticas.com/phpbb2/viewtopic.php?t=3122&highlight
28. http://www.costaricaticas.com/phpbb2/viewtopic.php?t=3122&highlight
29. http://www.costaricaticas.com/phpbb2/viewtopic.php?t=3122&highlight
30. http://www.costaricaticas.com/phpbb2/viewtopic.php?t=3122&highlight
31. http://www.costaricaticas.com/phpbb2/viewtopic.php?t=3401
32. http://www.costaricaticas.com/phpbb2/viewtopic.php?t=2706&highlight=poll
33. http://costaricasex.board.dk3.com/viewtopic.php?topic=644&forum=1&30

4. The sex worker

María gets dressed at her home in one of the working class neighborhoods that surround the capital city of San José. She works as a cashier during the day in Mas Por Menos, a large supermarket nearby. The area mushroom dwelling, where she lives, stretches for miles and miles towards the south and west of the capital. There are several large housing projects on the city's south side: parts of Desamparados and Pavas; Paso Ancho, San Sebastian, and of course, the eleven densely populated Hatillos. This sprawling district of San José began to develop back in the 1970's, thanks to housing plans drawn up by the National Housing and Urban Planning Institute (INVU), when the government was forced to accommodate the growing tide of rural migrants who began to inundate the cities, attracted by industrialization and the growth of the state apparatus. The President of Costa Rica at that time opposed birth control and roundly condemned family planning programs as a weapon of Yankee imperialism. This deluded politician believed that developed countries had an interest in maintaining Third World countries subjugated, as if strength lay in numbers. Nowadays he is involved in eco–tourism and complains of how the poor pollute his country especially the hotels he frequents.

Prosperity and the demands of an entrepreneurial and inefficient, corrupt state, did not necessarily reach everyone. And so, the area on the fringes of the city ended up with a name that is still uttered with a certain air of contempt: "the southern districts", though their inhabitants are not dispossessed but form a large part of Costa Rica's once thriving middle–class. Here you find everything: office workers, bank clerks, secretaries, university students and sex workers . . . as María. The woman makes the minimum wage at this supermarket, which amounts to $200 a month. "Not enough" She says, "to feed two children." María is not married and the two men who fathered her children, disappeared from her life several years ago. To make ends meet, she has another job at night. No one in her family or in her neighborhood knows about her second profession, one that allows her to make three times as much money as a cashier at the supermarket. María is a prostitute who services American male tourists and works in one of the trendiest nightclubs and hotels in San José. "My day job is only a front to make my neighbors think I make my money there," she tells us.

Sex workers, like María, are very different from their American clients. They are of different ethnic, linguistic, cultural, social, generational and religious backgrounds. (Tables 4–7)

According to our data from the 2000 survey, sex work is mostly an activity of very young women: 53% are younger than 29 years old; one third of them are younger than 24 years old; only one third are older than 35 years old.

Of the sex workers surveyed in 2000, 21% were then between 20 and 24 years old, and the oldest group, i.e. older than 40 years old, was 17% in 2000.

Most of the sex workers have not completed their secondary school: 23% have not finished primary school. Nevertheless, 92% do know how to read, and 89% know how to write. Very few of them (3%) have university studies. Notwithstanding these shortcomings, 58% have received training for a job.

The majority define themselves as Catholic (66%). One third of the sample considers themselves not very religious, and another third moderately religious.

Sex workers have a pattern of migrating from rural to urban areas. In the Metropolitan area of San José, 62% of the sex workers were born outside. 83% now live in it.

As for marital status, 57% of the sex workers are single, and 22% are cohabitating with a man. While 89% have children, only a very small minority is childless. Most of them have one or more than one dependants, and only 4% report zero dependants. With or without partners, these women bear the economic responsibility of home, especially of their own children.

Since the American tourist visits both the Massage Parlors and the nightclubs, these are the type of women who they will solicit sex work from. Nevertheless, many of them will only pick up the foreign women who work at the hotels for sex tourists. These women will be better educated, more urbanized and from better homes than the locals.

In Hotel Del Buey, almost 90% of the sex workers are foreigners. The major group is from Colombia, followed by sex workers from the Dominican Republic.

Foreign women play a very important role in Costa Rica's sex industry. The reason is that few of the women who engage in sex work in another country are sex workers at home. Migration allows mothers, wives, girlfriends, or daughters a high degree of anonymity and certain protection from discrimination at home while also protecting their family from being associated with a "loose" woman.[1]

According to our interviews, ethnographic observations and analysis of sex forums in the Internet, there are several reasons why these Colombian and

Dominican women control so much of the sex trade:

- They are professional. This means that, while in Costa Rica, they live off sex work exclusively and invest accordingly (breast implants, fitness club memberships, expensive clothing and perfumes). Being "pro" means they can be seen in restaurants, beach resorts, clubs and shopping malls with their clients. Costa Rican workers who live a double life and do sex work as a part time job, find it more difficult to be so exposed.
- They have a greater urban background. This translates into better "theater" in seduction and in pleasing American men than Costa Rican sex workers who are mainly from rural areas and thus shy away from certain sexual practices. Foreign sex workers also have a better command of English than Costa Rican sex workers.

Colombian and Dominican sex workers in Costa Rica have the same background as those in other Caribbean countries, such as in Panama, Curazao, Aruba, Haiti and Antigua. In 1996, 50,000 Dominican women were engaged in sex work outside the country, many of them worked regionally.[2] The reasons for engaging in sex work are not mainly abject poverty. A woman may run into a specific financial problem, and the idea that she can accumulate a large sum of money in a relatively short period of time through sex work often underlies a move into the trade. Many of these sex workers are formally known as small–scale entrepreneurs who travel outside the country to purchase merchandise to sell in their home territory and/or in other countries. Women often rely upon sex work to build up their initial capital in order to begin a trading career in household goods or other items. They tend to leave sex work once the capital is accumulated.

The women work abroad to escape from the whore stigma. This is a powerful discourse that both dishonors and controls, in particular but not exclusively, female sexuality. As in the case of the Dominican Republic, it creates a climate where certain forms of sex work are met with intense disapproval. Even in places where prostitution is partially legalized, as in Curazao, the stigma has a profound effect.[3] The majority of Colombian and Dominican sex workers has obtained a secondary level of education, was engaged in semiskilled occupations or business when not in sex work, and came from urban centers.[4]

The women come to this country mostly on their own and through recommendations by other sex workers. Most of them are not under the control of pimps or trafficking agencies and the stay in the country is usually for a year; many stay longer and travel back and forth to their native country. Their main objective is to save money to start a business back home or in Costa Rica. They also send money to their families back home. It is important to note that the amounts sent home by Caribbean migrants constitute a large and important part of national incomes. In the Dominican Republic during the 1980's, for example, remittances amounted to about one–fourth of the country's foreign currency. [5]

A smaller group of sex workers are indeed trafficked to Costa Rica by regional agencies that advance money to them and withdraw their passports until the debts are fully paid. According to Casa Alianza, the trafficking includes women from several countries, such as the Dominican Republic, Colombia, the Philippines, Panama and Europe. [6]

Casa Alianza provides the means used by these agencies to recruit women for sex work: They look for people who are poor, place advertisements in local newspapers, offer job opportunities and good salaries, the opportunity to travel; establish fraudulent business and travel agencies; contract fake marriages to lure young women; and take advantage of soft laws against trafficking. [7]

Social status

A survey of material goods owned by the women shows that 84% of the sex workers have color T.V, 72% have a refrigerator, 69% own a washing machine, 20% have a microwave oven, an a third own a VHS. Other items such as telephones (11%), computers (4.5%), and cars (6.0%) are less available. (Table 5) Ownership of such items indicates sex workers are not poor, nor they come from the lowest social backgrounds. In Costa Rican standards, they are mostly middle–class. While many women in the US and other countries become sex workers because of drug and alcohol addictions, rarely is that the case in Costa Rica (with the exception of the streetwalkers). Most sex workers in Costa Rica are there to better their economic situations and care for their families. Some will work only a few days per month, while others make it a career choice. You will find women from Nicaragua, Argentina, Venezuela, Russia, Romania, Colombia, Dominican Republic and even Nevada, USA, working the streets, bars and clubs of San José.

It is evident that prices have increased in the last five years and, consequently, so have the incomes of sex workers. The ones that work inside the sexual tourism industry have higher incomes than the ones shown in the surveys. In Hotel Del Buey, for example, the cost for one hour can range from $100 to $500 depending on the 'characteristics' of the sexual worker. Between the sale of liquor and the price from the sexual exchange, the women that are deemed the most attractive can earn around $1,000 to $2,000 per night. Mexpat knows that "high quality poontang in the Del Buey can get expensive."

"More and more chicas are asking $100 an hour firm and some are coming off the top with $200 or $300 for a few hours or *toda la noche*." The reason, according to him is because "Unfortunately a lot of tourists are paying these prices which is just aggravating the problem." The solution he sees is to look for cheaper street sex workers: "Yes, there are still lots of very fine chicas who will go for $50 or 20,000 *colones*." The only problem is to find them: "locating the ones who will go for this and give great service is tricky."[8]

Depending on their sexual appeal, some women are able to charge more than that. There is a famous TV star, for example, which is able to demand $7,000 per night. But this is an exception. The majority will negotiate their prices but only a few will go down to less than $80 an hour. With these rates, many sex workers can pocket around $500 per night. The average income is around $2,000 a week, not bad for a country where a professional makes around $500 a month.

Girls who work at massage parlors are not so lucky. The average income in MP 6 –based on three clients a day– is around $1,600 a month. CapoD2 makes the following calculations on their earnings.

> *NOW lets sum up situation 3 of burnout and for arguments sake let us use MP 6. By no means are these #'s accurate just a broad spectrum.*
> *Girl works 6 days a week 3 weeks out of the month because of her Cycle. Throw in 2 more days during the cycle front back that's 20 days per month.*
> *20 Days Per month!*
> *Average amount of encounters 3 per day!*
> *1?2 of House Take Averaging in CRT discounts $22.00 per encounter.*
> *Tips per encounter Highs, Lows and Stiffs (No Pun) $5.00 per encounter*
> *That's 27.00 per session x 3 per day x 20 days or $1620.00 per month, give or take..NOT BAD in fact let us also take into account that's great money for CR.*

But CapoD2 recognizes later on that perhaps this is not such a great income:

> *Top 10 Reasons for Burnout making that Kind of Money!*
>
> *10. She has to take 6–10 showers per day one before, one after, one before she gets to work, one after.*
> *9. She has to put her make up on 4–5 Times per day.*
> *8. She has to take average 2 Steams or Saunas per day.*
> *7. She has to give 3 massages per day!*
> *6. She has to entice you to a session and smile and be nice all day in the waiting room.*
> *5. She has to try to have a real relationship, and have sex with her novio and act excited about after she has been doing all of the items below.*
> *4. She has to act all enthused giving BBBJ's all day to Fat overweight Drkkunk, hung–over, gringos.*
> *3. She has to kiss Fat overweight Drunk, hung–over, gringos.*

2. *She gets to be fondled all day by Fat overweight Drunk, hung–over, gringos.*
1. *She has to have enthusiastic sex all day with Fat overweight Drunk, hung–over, gringos.*

Maybe $1620.00 per month isn't that much after all! [9]

Sex workers from Casa Mila and many other places do not make that much money. Contrary to the $100 asking price at Hotel Del Buey, women here charge ten times less. [10]

Sex workers who cater to tourists are making more money than the average Costa Rican doctor, lawyer, University professor or even the President of the country. Theses incomes, in theory, put them at the top of the income ladder. A look less rosy when you investigate the sex worker's spending habits. One of them is the woman's contribution to her home. María, for example, has to support her two children plus her mother, two sisters and two nieces. She pays their rent and also the children's education. Lupe supports her four brothers and her ailing father. Cristina pays her mother's medical costs and also her sister who is mentally challenged. Another large expense goes on their clothes and make–up. Sex workers who work for the American tourist cannot look cheap. They must buy their clothes at expensive boutiques and do their hair at the most sophisticated hair salons. Shoes, perfumes, jewelry and purses are also expensive. They also pay lots of money in transportation, as they need to use the discreet taxi driver who hides them from the public. Additionally, sex workers spend lots of money in gambling, drugs and alcohol. The ones who work in the "*fichaje*" system are heavily addicted to crack and booze. Once you take all these expenses into account, plus the very short period of attractiveness (18 to 25 years old), the average sex worker does not live any better than the Latin American lower middle class.

Notes

1. Kamala Kempadoo, *Sexing the Caribbean. Gender, Race, and Sexual Labor*, London: Routledge, 2004 , ebook, pp. 2187–2188.
2. IOM Migraton Information Programme, "Trafiking in Women from the Dominican Republic for Sexual Exploitation" (Geneva: International Organization on Migration, 1996).
3. Kamala Kempadoo, *Sexing the Caribbean. Gender, Race, and Sexual Labor*, London: Routledge, 2004 , ebook, p.2190.
4. Kamala Kempadoo, *Sexing the Caribbean. Gender, Race, and Sexual Labor*, London: Routledge, 2004 , ebook, p.2301

5. Kamala Kempadoo, *Sexing the Caribbean. Gender, Race, and Sexual Labor,* London: Routledge, 2004 , ebook, p.2305.

6. *Sex Tourism: A Contributing Factor to the Trafficking of Persons in Latin America,* in www.worldsexguide.com

7. Ibid.

8. http://www.costaricaticas.com/phpbb2/viewtopic.php?t=1483

9. http://www.costaricaticas.com/phpbb2/viewtopic.php?t=2615

10. http://www.costaricaticas.com/phpbb2/viewtopic.php?t=1483

5. HIV in the Caribbean and Central America.

The Caribbean, according to Kempadoo, "defies static definition." It is a region constituted through a violent history of Spanish, British, Dutch, French and Danish conquest, settlement, and colonial rule that involved the genocide of the indigenous peoples as well as the forced importation of million of African slaves. [1] It is constituted by countries that range from Haiti, the first black republic to declare its independence in 1804, to Suriname and Belize, which gained independence during the last quarter of the twentieth century. In some instances it is defined only by the islands– the Antilles (Greater and Lesser, Dutch, French, and British). Other times it includes territories washed by the Caribbean Sea– the Circum Caribbean coastlands of Central and South America or *El Caribe* Insular. Throughout this flux of definitions, the Spanish–speaking territories– Cuba, the Dominican Republic, Puerto Rico, and the "Caribbean" regions of Colombia, Venezuela and Suriname– have been included and excluded, sometimes isolated from the rest of the region as parts of Latin America [2] In the current UN structure, as well as that of regional political and economic organizations, the "Caribbean" excludes Central America and Colombia. This means that epidemiological studies and prevention interventions on HIV follow arrangements –that more often than not– don't follow the patterns of regional sex tourism. Costa Rica, for example, is included in Central America; the Dominican Republic in the Spanish Caribbean, and Colombia in South America. Nevertheless, both sex workers and sex tourists do not follow this arrangement, as the patterns of travel are influenced more by race and airline connections rather than geography. American and local tourists, as Kempadoo indicates, fly mainly to the Dominican Republic, Colombia and Costa Rica on the basis of the phenotype characteristics of the women (lighter skinned) rather than because of political or geographical considerations.

By reinvoking race here, I am insisting that historical social and processes and constructs that created social difference in terms of phenotype and ethnicity in the Caribbean continue to shape and inform social relations in the twenty–first century, despite the lack of single, homogenous, region–wide discourse on the subject, and in spite of the often–heard claims that racism no longer exists in the region. [3]

An estimated 1.9 million adults and children are living with HIV in this area. Twelve countries in this region, including the Dominican Republic and Haiti, several Central American countries (such as Belize and Honduras), and Guyana and Suriname, have an estimated HIV prevalence of 1% or more among pregnant women. In several Caribbean countries, adult HIV prevalence rates are surpassed only by the rates experienced in sub–Saharan Africa—making this the second–most affected region in the world. Recent projections for El Salvador, Guatemala, and Panama done with the Spectrum Model indicate that the epidemic could reach adult prevalence levels of close to 2% in these countries by 2010 on current patterns. [4]

Throughout the world, the unequal social status of women places them at higher risk for contracting HIV. Women are at a disadvantage when it comes to access to information about HIV prevention, the ability to negotiate safe sexual encounters, and access to treatment for HIV/AIDS once infected. In accordance with these inequities, the HIV infection rate among women is rising faster than the infection rate among men in the Caribbean and Latin America. [5]

The epidemic is spreading to an increasing proportion of women. Infection rates are generally highest in the cities and major economic areas. In San Pedro Sula, Honduras, for example, HIV infection hovers between 2–5% in pregnant women. [6] The primary mode of transmission is unprotected sex. Female sex workers are at risk, with infection rates of 0.3 percent to 10.3 percent (0.6 percent in Nicaragua, 1.9 percent in Panama, 3.9 percent in El Salvador, 4.6 percent in Guatemala, and 10.3 percent in Honduras). Clients of commercial sex workers act as a bridge between high–risk groups and the general population, including foreign tourists. [7] (Table 22)

Women's risk is further exacerbated because they are physiologically 2 to 4 times more susceptible to HIV. Women have a larger mucosal surface where micro–lesions can occur. Young girls and adolescents, whose reproductive tracts are not fully developed, are even more susceptible to STIs and HIV. Untreated STIs increase women's risk of HIV infection. Women who have been coerced into unprotected sex or raped are more likely to be infected with HIV since rough, forced sex causes more lesions in vaginal and anal tissues. [8] Studies have also shown that girls and boys who are victims of physical and/or sexual abuse during childhood are more likely to exhibit high–risk sexual behavior later in life, and decreased ability to negotiate safer sex due to lowered self–esteem. [9] Because many of the women enter countries illegally and commercial sex is usually illegal, they are not protected by law, experience social stigma, and have almost no access to social and medical services. [10] Not having access to health and medical care, counseling, and information means that they are less likely to receive accurate prognosis and treatment of HIV. [11]

Sex workers living with HIV are often stigmatized, leading to the loss of housing, employment, denial of health care and insurance, and rejection by family and community. The stigma surrounding HIV/AIDS causes most of them to choose not to be tested

Central America has a history of intraregional and extra regional migration due to civil unrest, demand for seasonal labor, more open border policies, improved regional transportation routes, and proximity to the United States. The unstable economic environment provoked by Hurricane Mitch in 1998, combined with uneven growth and employment prospects in individual countries, have further increased mobility, including that of sex workers. Sex tourist destinations such as Costa Rica have large populations of illegal Central American and Caribbean sex workers.

Despite increased awareness of HIV/AIDS, senior policymakers outside of the health sector in many Central American countries have not yet integrated HIV/AIDS prevention into ongoing policy and programmatic activities.

The Costa Rican epidemic

The most recent statistics provided by the Health Ministry registered a total of 2,357 AIDS patients in Costa Rica as of July 31, 2002 (*Tico Times*, Nov. 28, 2003). According to UNAIDS, there is a low estimate of adults and children (6,000) with AIDS and a high estimate of 21,000 (it includes HIV infections and full–blown AIDS). Women have a low estimate of 2,000 and a high of 6,600. Since 1985, 1,528 Costa Ricans are known to have died of AIDS–related complications. UNAIDS provides a low estimate of 400 AIDS–related deaths in 2003 and a high of 1,600. [12]

Though the Health Ministry's official numbers indicate 110 new cases of the illness in 2003, up from 90 in 2002, the AIDS Control Office of the Ministry told AFP newswire it records nearly 450 cases per year. Public hospitals reportedly receive 450 new AIDS patients per year, but the Health Ministry only has recorded a quarter of those cases and Ministry representatives say its statistics are the only ones that are considered official.

Chavarría, from the AIDS Control Office, said it is disturbing that the percentage of infected women in Costa Rica has risen from 7% of the total in the early 1990s to 20% of the total today. The trend is of an increased risk for women. In the latest report from the *Caja Costarricense del Seguro Social*, Costa Rica's social medicine agency, in the first 26 weeks of 2004, the number of new HIV and STI cases in the Metropolitan Area are almost the same for men and women. That signifies an increase of the epidemic among the heterosexual population and an expected increase in cases of infected newborns.

According to members of an AIDS support group in San José many women contract the disease from their husbands who have unprotected sex with others.[13]

Sex workers

Official statistics on sex workers and HIV in Costa Rica are scant. We only have data that indicate that the infection rate among sex workers increased from 0.4% in 1992 to 0.6% in 1994 to 0.8% in 1995. [14] The last report revealed that the infection rate is less than 5%. Nevertheless, this data is based on registered prostitutes from very low socioeconomic background. According to this report, there were 3,920 new infections during 2003, of which 523 were female and 72 belong to sex workers (13.8%). [15] The number of HIV–infected sex workers who work for the tourist industry is unknown.

In a small country such as Costa Rica given the evidence we have on unsafe sex in the sex industry, 100 sex workers who are HIV positive can have a large impact on the monger population. These men repeatedly share the same sex workers who do not always use condoms. Despite this threat many of the "experts" on HIV and Costa Rica's monger community –such as Prolijo– still think that AIDS is not a major concern. Prolijo thinks the articles on HIV and sex work in Central America are rather pessimistic:

> *I don't want to gloss over this report because AIDS is serious business, but I would like to point out a few ameliorating factors and some tips. First, the current 0.55% HIV/AIDS infection rate is still very low compared to many other countries . . . Second, notice the subgroups with the highest rates of infection –gays, prisoners (presumably due to gay sex), the Afro–Caribbean groups, street Children and yes also CSW's. My guess is that, as in the US, this problem is more serious among the lower class sex workers such as street walkers, which most of us don't frequent, and lower class brothels, which some of us do...The reason I am guessing it is also more prevalent in the lower class brothels is that they are frequented more heavily by men who are not as educated about the perils of AIDS or refuse to wear them as part of their culture (ie brothels that cater more to Ticos). So my advice is don't use street walkers or local brothels. There is also overlap of gays, Afro–Carib and CSW in the Caribbean*

port towns of Limon and Puerto Viejo and I am sure the AIDS/HIV rate is highest in that part of CR, bringing up the country's average rate. So my second piece of advice is don't go to the Atlantic coast for sex. I realize that there are also some among us who go to the local brothels or who still go bare for genital to genital sex, so we still shouldn't ignore this problem, but I think the risk is far less amongst the BM girls most of whom see only 1–2 clients per day if that and who, although they provide BBBJ's, usually insist on a condom for the actual deed...
This article just fits into the alarmist campaign of the CR government and US religious groups against the sex trade. Perhaps, I am sticking my head into the sand on this issue, but I think distinctions must be made between various subgroups within the sex market. We are not all pedophiles, or gay or go with IV drug–using streetwalkers, or high–volume low rent local brothels. [16]

Others, such as Kotigre, think there are no STIs to worry about in Costa Rica: "I never use a condom and I never heard of any STDs in CR so I wouldn't worry. By the way, I've got these perpetual blisters that keep coming back on and around my lips. Anybody knows if it's because I'm not getting enough sun and vitamin C?" [17]

Depending on the source, we have two different stories on STI statistics. The number of new STI, according to the official reports of the Ministry of Health, is increasing but not an alarming rate. The number of gonorrhea cases, for example, rose from 1,278 in 2001 to 1,847 in 2003. Syphilis, on the other hand, remains stable and urethritis of the non–gonorrhea type shows a light increase from 2001 to 2003. The number of AIDS' new cases in 2003 is almost half of the number in the year 2000. (Tables 23–24)

If we only relied on the Ministry of Health's reports for our HIV information, the picture of the epidemic seems very optimistic. There are fewer AIDS' new cases and the epidemic seems to be in decline since the year 2000. Nevertheless, another picture arises from the hospitals' data. This information is more reliable because it comes from the diagnosis made at the places where most Costa Ricans are treated and not from a bureaucratic department that requires doctors to report the new HIV cases.

Hospitals report four times more new AIDS cases than the Ministry of Health. This means more than 450 new AIDS cases a year.

The difference in numbers can be explained by the fear many doctors at public hospitals have of reporting the true diagnosis to the Ministry, a practice that makes perfect sense in a society with little tradition of confidentiality.

If we add to this number the AIDS' patients treated in private clinics and hospitals, the reality of the AIDS epidemic in Costa Rica might look very different and perhaps duplicates the one suggested by the public hospitals.

The situation in the hospitals is a drastic increase in STIs and HIV among the general population and among sex workers. [18] The country's HIV infection rate is becoming similar to Thailand's since the data indicates 1% sero prevalence among the heterosexual population, 6% among homosexuals and 8% sero prevalence among bisexuals.

- Congenital syphilis shows a progressive increase from 1994 to 2001.
- Between 1993 and 2002, there are 98 new cases of congenital syphilis per year.
- 7 of each 100 heterosexuals has syphilis and one has HIV
- 7 of each homosexual men have syphilis and 6 are HIV+
- 9 of 100 bisexual men have syphilis and 8 are HIV+
- 55 of 100 registered sex workers have bacterial *vaginosis*

Contrary to some of the monger's optimism about HIV in Costa Rica, this data suggests that the epidemic is a serious threat to both the American and the Costa Rican communities.

Notes

1. Kamala Kempadoo, *Sexing the Caribbean. Gender, Race, and Sexual Labor.* London: Rooutledge, 2004, ebook edition.

2. Kamala Kempadoo, *Sexing the Caribbean. Gender, Race, and Sexual Labor.* London: Rooutledge, 2004, ebook edition, p. 148–150.

3. Kamala Kempadoo, *Sexing the Caribbean. Gender, Race, and Sexual Labor.* London: Rooutledge, 2004, ebook edition, p. 145.

4. PASCA, Spectrum Model, 2002.

5. Women and HIV/AIDS, WHO Fact sheet 242 (2000) http://www.who.int/inf–fs/en/fact242.html. AIDS Epidemic Update, UNAIDS/WHO (2004)

6. UNAIDS, Fact Sheet 2002: Latin American and the Caribbean, 2002.

7. AIDS – 5 years since ICPD, UNAIDS (1999) http://www.unaids.org/publications/documents/human/gender/newsletter.pdf

8. Ending Violence Against Women" Population Reports 27(4). JHUCCP (1999) http://www.jhuccp.org/pr/l11edsum.stm

9. If Not Now, When? Addressing Gender–Based Violence in Refugee, Internally Displaced and Post–Conflict Settings. Reproductive Health for Refugees Consortium (2002) http://www.rhrc.org/resources/gbv/wc_gbvcontents.html

10. Gender and HIV/AIDS UNAIDS Fact Sheet (2001) http://www.unaids.org/fact_sheets/files/GenderFS_en.pdf

11. Costa Rica. Epidemiological Fact Sheets on HIV/Aids and Sexually Transmitted Infections, UNAIDS, 2004, P.2.

12. Tico Times, Feb 27, 2004

13. Epidemiological Fact Sheets on HIV/AIDS and Sexually Transmitted Infections

Costa Rica 2002 Update, UNAIDS 2002.

14. Costa Rica. Epidemiological Fact Sheets on HIV/Aids and Sexually Transmitted Infections, UNAIDS, 2004, P.2.

15. http://www.costaricaticas.com/phpbb2/viewtopic.php?t=718

16. http://www.costaricaticas.com/phpbb2/viewtopic.php?t=3928

17. The Tico Times, Weekly Edition: Vol. VIII, No. 131, August 27 2004.

6. Sexual practices

Jeff, who sat next to Lorna in the American Airlines' flight to San José, took a taxi to Hotel Del Buey after going through immigration at Santamaría's Airport. He had reserved his hotel room three months in advance and upon arriving threw his small suitcase on his single bed and took the elevator downstairs to the Blue Queen, the hotel's bar. María was sitting on a bar stool and greeted him warmly as she needed to make some cash. After exchanging some words in Spanglish, the couple decided to have sex. Jeff payed $10 extra at the hotel's Reception for having a "visitor" in his room, checked María in, and eloped upstairs. They both agreed to have sex and the price agreed was $100 for the hour. According to Jeff, price negotiation was the hardest part of the deal. According to María, sexual practice is the most difficult part of her job. "What do you mean by that?"-we inquired. "It is the Gringos demands that sometimes drives me crazy," she says.

If you studied the sexual abbreviations in the most visited sex forums on Costa Rica, you would find a large repertoire of sexual practices.

Bareback– Without a condom.
BBBJ– Bareback Blow Job, oral stimulation of the penis without a condom
BBBJTC–Bareback Blow Job to Completion, oral stimulation of the penis to orgasm without a condom. (May spit or swallow)
BS&TL'er: Ball Sucking & Taint Licking -(For those of you who may not be aware of this area of the male anatomy), the "taint" was named for the small sensitive area under the scrotum. I was told about this zone by an old military buddy of mine from Louisiana . . . . He said the area was so named "cuz it Taint your nuts & it Taint your ass.)"
Cash and Dash– A rip–off. She shows up, takes your money, doesn't provide, might offer to "dance", and leaves.
CBJCBJ– Covered Blow Job, fellatio with a condom

CFS – Covered Full Service.
CIM– Cum in mouth.
Clock–watcher– A term for a provider who counts the minutes until the session is over. Usually used to describe a provider who rushes and does not enjoy her work.
Completion Orgasm. E.g. she gave a bareback blowjob to completion.
Cowgirl Woman rides on top, knees astride.
DATY Dining at the Y– Cunnilingus, oral stimulation of the vulva or clitoris.
DFK– Deep French Kissing, kissing with tongue
FOTC– Phuck of the century.
French– Oral sex, on party
FS Full Service– Vaginal intercourse to completion
GFE Girl Friend Experience– A subjective term, but usually used as praise for a very passionate, sensual, non–mechanical experience. Most consider deep French kissing a baseline requirement for GFE.
Greek– Anal Sex
LFK– Light French kissing. (No heavy tongue)
NQBS Non–quitter, but spitter – BBBJTC and spits your ejaculate.
NQNS Non–quitter, non–spitter– BBBJTC and swallows your ejaculate.
PSE Porn Star Experience– A subjective term, used as praise for a provider that might have a high energy level, a particularly hot look, or is very accommodating ("nastiness" factor).
Reverse Cowgirl– woman rides on top, facing away
Spinner a very petite provider. Etymology: From the 1970's toy, "Sit 'n' Spin"[1]

Despite the broad sexual menu, there are culturally different interpretations for similar sexual acts.

María told us, for example, that the aboe list was not descriptive of the what actually happens in the bedroom. She said that the first lesson she learned when having sex with American partners was the "never ending desire for oral sex." In her sexual practices with Latino men, she added, "oral sex is less important." "Some years ago, she continued, most clients did not care that much about it. It is American porno movies and tourists that have brought the trend." María, as a sex worker, would like to finish her client as soon as possible and masturbation and vaginal sex is according to her "the techniques that do the trick faster." But in the case of oral sex, "it is harder to make them come and I have to do all the work"- she complained.

For the Costa Rican sex worker, oral sex is not part of the traditional sexual practice. Latin men –according to María– are more into anal sex and into large and rounded butts. Large breasts are not such a strong turn–on as they are for the American male tourist. As a matter of fact, the rush of sex workers to have breast implants is a result more of American tastes than from local demand. The sex workers with silicone breasts are easily recognized as targeting the American market. Nevertheless, the Americans, as the self–poll taken at costaricaticas.com indicates, are not turned on by silicone breasts.[2] Despite the American taste for the "natural grown", many can not tell whether the women have had or not the operation, something that makes the professional sex worker decide to go for surgery.

According to the members of the sex forum, anal sex is also not liked by sex workers. Nevertheless, if more money is provided, it is not rejected. Badboy, for example, asks what percentage of women like anal sex. Prolijo responds that it is not popular but "I'm sure some would take it if you offered enough dinero." Administrator 3 indicates that "the vast majority of Ticas are not into Greek, but if you are looking for it, to try the Nicaraguan sex workers."[3]

Sex workers have control over their minds and bodies through different interpretations of sexual practices. Oral and anal sex and French kissing are perceived as intimate, something to be done only to please a "novio" or a lover. When Americans demand oral sex as an important part of the repertoire, they are asking for something not provided in commercial sex. The sex worker resist by asking for extra money or by doing it without passion, something that makes the client feel ripped off.

Many sex workers, on the other hand, perceive condoms as a barrier to intimacy. American men do not understand why sex workers ask them whether or not they want to use condoms. They fail to comprehend –as it will be analyzed later– the emotional implications of having unprotected sex.

Sex tourists have their own favorite sexual practices and sometimes have problems in being satisfied. One of the major attractions is deep or French kissing. Joe1015, for example, said that his number one rule is "lots of French kissing since making love without lots of kissing is like eating food without seasoning."[4] Despite the strong liking for this sexual practice, many men complain that "some of the women do not like French kissing. Astroglide, for example, revealed that some of the women avoid it. For him, "besos is a major part of the turn on. I never even give that a second thought." To prevent problems, bad breath and mouth infections, he "brings a bottle of Listerine and do a lot of washouts on my trips." Nevertheless, "The biggest challenge is not IF I should kiss her, but finding one that really LOVES to make out." This "sometimes is a challenge." "Nothing turns me off more than a babe that seems hot downstairs, and then when I get her upstairs she turns her head and offers the cheek, or purses her lips."[5]

As sexual practices become loaded with different perceptions of intimacy, so does HIV prevention. Sex workers find it easier to prevent French kissing than vaginal sex without a condom. María, for example, confessed that she had more problems kissing customers than in letting them penetrate her: "I only kiss my lover. I don´t let customers touch my tongue, this is only done when you are in love." When we asked her whether vaginal sex is less intimate for her, she answered that "it is not so close to me because I don´t see neither his penis nor my vagina, both are too down below."

On the other hand, customers are stricter with regard to having vaginal sex without a condom in their non–regular relationships. Nevertheless, they do not mind taking some risks when practicing oral sex. Most of them like to practice *cunnilungus* and are aware that there are some risks involved. This is also the case with French kissing and breast milk. Hotluck advises others never to "brush your teeth prior to Oral Ops. Can cause micro tears of the gums, mouth lining. Could be an infective path."- He says. He does not advise to brush after and suggests gargling. "Less stress on the mouth. Something high in alcohol content. Listerine or Scotch, your flavor." He knows, nevertheless, the majority will take their chances and each one should decide "what your personal risk tolerance is and then go do those things." His final thought is not to worry that much and to "Have fun."[6]

Carla, a sex worker, thinks that mongers are very naive in their behavior: "I sometimes have four or five clients a night. Some do not want to use a condom and are willing to pay more for it. Others, such as the older guys, love to lick my clitoris and vagina and spend a good time in this. One or two have bleeding gums or constantly brush their teeth before and after the act. Sometimes I am able to clean myself between customers, but in other times, I don't have neither the time nor the facilities to do so. I don´t understand why they are so conscious about using condoms for vaginal sex but don´t protect themselves with regard to oral sex."

Finally, mongers are also aware that both the client and the sex workers are at risk when practicing oral sex. Jazz Musician recognizes that sex workers themselves do not know the risks they engage with their customers: "I'm telling ya, you can't trust these phuckin' mongers, especially V–Bob. His D*ck has been everywhere!" They obviously cannot tell either the risks the women engage in: "Seriousness aside, you don't know where that honey next to you in an American bar has been either. Take her out to dinner first. Unless she performs a quickie in the men's room while you're looking at the menu, you should be safe."[7]

Notes

1. http://www.costaricaticas.com/phpbb2/viewtopic.php?t=1774
2. http://www.costaricaticas.com/phpbb2/viewtopic.php?t=1774
3. http://www.costaricaticas.com/phpbb2/viewtopic.php?t=1774

4. http://www.costaricaticas.com/phpbb2/viewtopic.php?t=4183
5. http://www.costaricaticas.com/phpbb2/viewtopic.php?t=4183
6. http://www.costaricaticas.com/phpbb2/viewtopic.php?t=4183
7. http://www.costaricaticas.com/phpbb2/viewtopic.php?t=4183

7. Condom use

The Women

According to a PAHO (Pan American Health Organization) report, "Commercial sex workers in Central America are at high risk of HIV infection because their customers frequently do not use condoms. Sex workers often do not insist on the use of condoms since they underestimate the risk of infection, they do not have access to condoms, or they earn more money by providing unprotected sex. Clients of sex workers act as a bridge between high–risk groups and the general population."[1]

In our 2000 survey, unsafe sex was high and 40% of the sample had practiced vaginal sex without a condom during the last year; 9% of the sample practiced anal sex without a condom; 14% had oral sex with ejaculation without a condom. (Table 10)

We see different self–taken polls and postings from chat rooms about condom use with sex workers. In the most recent one carried in 2005, almost 50% of the mongers admitted having had sex with sex workers without a condom.

Have you ever had bbfs[2] in CR with intent[3], within the past 3 years?

Yes	49%	[45]
No	50%	[46]
	Total Votes:	91[4]

Papichulo, for example, had a fiasco in his trip: "My last trip we had sex a few times sin condom, she claimed to be on the pill, but now says that the antibiotics she was on for a foot injury made the pill null & void." According to him, "Drunken moments happen" and this time "she's pregnant." Papichulo is desperate and asks for help to his fellow mongers: "She quickly became my novia (whether I wanted it or not). ! Slipped in . . . felt so good . . . she didnt stop me . . . so it was off to the races! God damn am I am idiot!"[5]

His friends tell him not to trust the woman until a DNA test is done. Nevertheless, if the child turns to be his, he has obligations because part of the relationship is "to take care of the *novia.*"[6]

Witling warns other mongers that most sex workers asked him to have sex without a condom. He admits being "shocked at the number of girls who wanted to Phuck me bareback." Nevertheless, of the women he was with "I must have had about 8 different girls who requested that I take off the condom. I felt like grabbing them by the shoulders and shaking the shit out of them. 'Do you know how dangerous that is? You don't know what I might have, you should never Phuck without a condom!!"

Despite Witling's strong stand in favor of prevention and his rejection of unsafe sex, he himself recognizes to have being tempted and ready to submit: "I have to be honest and say I was really tempted with a couple of them, especially 2 girls."[7] Prolijo, on the other hand, thinks it takes two to tango. In a discussion over how many porno stars haven been infected, he sees a parallel with mongers. He asks: "How many of them take them up on the offer? How many of them try to pressure the girls to perform other unsafe practices that they don't want to?" Many take their chances, he says and "This is a story of the risks we ALL face if we have unprotected sex with a untested sex worker. Guys go bareback in the porn biz so that viewers can enjoy the "money shot". We don't have to do that and there is no reason why we should take any unnecessary risks." Notwithstanding his admonitions, he knows that "When I read this thread, I can only shake my own shoulders and say, "some people never learn".[8]

Joe1015 admits he never used condoms for oral sex at the Massage Parlor. He also indicates that he was offered the same for vaginal sex. "Never wore a condom at MP 6 for BJ.I was even asked with or without when it came to penetration, and I chose to get some coverage. Maybe this can help."[9] Jack52 is afraid of having gotten infected from unprotected sex. He feels sorry now but it is too late. "Had unprotected sex, with a seasoned *puta*. Did not go down on her, kissed and had two sessions. Had been a good boy for a few weeks prior to doing her. I want her to be tested if possible, boy was i stupid!!"[10]

Goetzvonberlishingen wondered whether sex workers are tested since they generally practice unsafe sex. "I had a session at MP 6 last trip during which the *chica*, who is quite popular on this board asked me if I wanted to use a condom for the main sex part. I was a little shocked and said yes, but I am wondering if these MP girls are routinely going bareback for the main deal. That gives me a little concern over the safety situation. Anyone else experience this?"[11]

Goetz explained that sex workers have bareback sex as a sign of trust and intimacy. "I just return from CR last week and a girl that I was with all night about 4 times when I was there asked me if I would like to have sex *sin condom*? (We used a condom all the other times) I declined, but I took as a sign of trust and she being comfortable with me."[12] The same happened to Goetz who admitted being asked by the women at the MP's to have unsafe sex: "During my last trip, out of all the sessions I had at ZB I also had one that asked for sex sin condom. Of course I denied her and told her con condom, but it also surprised me a little, especially coming from a MP *chica* who sees numerous clients a day. In the end though I did CIM as a compromise."[13]

Condoms in trash cans

There are other means to inquire into the realities of unsafe sex. We counted the number of condoms in trashcans in the most popular massage parlors (Tuesday, October 13, 2004; from open to closing hours) The results are listed bellow:

Massage Parlor	Number of clients	Number of condoms
MP 2	25	11
MP 3	40	27
MP 4	20	9

We cannot tell how many times each client had sex with one or more sex workers. We also cannot know the sexual practices clients engaged in. It is a fact that many of them do not consider oral sex without a condom as unsafe sex. Perhaps many of them do not practice vaginal or anal penetration, the riskiest practices for HIV infection. Nevertheless, it is evident that condoms are not used in around 50% of the time.

For sex workers the main reason for not using condoms is money. In the massage parlors, sex workers have different prices for "bareback" sex. Lila, who works at MP4, charges $50 with a condom and $100 without it. Dildoman recognizes that some mongers pay up to $200 per session. He thinks this is too much money and also too unwise.

He said, "yeah but I can do anything I want with these girls".
I replied, "you mean anal sex?"
He said. "no dude, I can screw them without a condom!"
Not a very smart guy.[14]

From 1997 to 2000 some NGO's and a program from Social Marketing of Condoms (PASMO) carried out workshops on prevention and on the correct use of condom to sex workers from the low–income sector in Costa Rica. Despite these interventions, the results were poor. It was found, for example, in the 2000 Survey (Table 19) very low grades in our battery of steps to observe correct condom use:

> *Twenty–seven per cent of the respondents opened their condoms with their teeth. Only 3% checked for the expiration date. Only twenty–four per cent cheked for air bubbles.*
>
> *If we take into account those who correctly opened the condom with their fingers in one corner, those who squeezed the tip of the condom to expel air, and those who correctly unrolled the condom to cover the dildo, we have that only 18% passed the test.*
>
> *If we add into consideration those who held the ring of the condom when pulling the condom out of the dildo, the index drops to 11%.*
>
> *The index drops even lower when we take into account the 9 variables selected to analyze proper condom use. Only 0.5% of the sample succeeded.*

The situation must be very serious with sex workers who exclusively work with tourists since they are not registered by the Ministry of Health and do not receive any health education.

You would expect the American tourist to be knowledgeable of condoms and at ease with them. We do not know their ability to use them properly, but we do find lots of anxiety about buying them. Older men buying condoms is something that is not so well accepted in the States and mongers feel ridiculed for it. This suggests that there might be possible difficulties when talking about them and using them with sex workers. Bombero, for example, buys condoms in the Internet since he does not like to be seen shopping for them at regular stores: "Thank goodness for the internet because I really hate buying those things in stores." [15] Twarag sympathizes with Bombero since he also gets questioned from clerks at Eckerd why a man his age is buying condoms: "Last month she laughingly said that your prescription order reflects a man of a certain age but the rest of my order gives a different story. Told her I am active and she laughed and agreed." [16] Carib_ Wanderer reports to get weird looks from the cashier at Target.

> *Last trip I bought my 36–pack of rubbers at Target, along with 20 small bottles of body wash and lotions, bottle of K–Y, 15 of those hair clips that the chicas keep clipped on their purses, 12 shower caps (chicas love those), and lots of hershey's kisses (they love those too). The cashier was looking at me like I was*

from Mars; she probably was thinking "what the hell???" [17]

Phat Prophet also reports nasty looks at Walmart once the condoms and the women's conditioners are seen at the cashier's.

> *Last time I got to go to Cuba I was stocking up, girl at the checkout noticed all the meds and sun screen and asked if I was going on a trip. I said yes and she was real chatty till she grabbed the xtra large box of condoms and after that a few dozen little bottles of shampoo and conditioner and stuff like that. She wasnt nearly as friendly after those items. Wonder why? Hehe.* [18]

Mongers also experiment with non–latex condoms, which lead them to take serious risks. [19] Some are aware that there are risks involved, but engaged in them anyway. Goetzvonberlishingen, for example, is aware that these condoms are not FDA– approved and have greater risks for tears or breaks. He has not had problems with the condoms; nevertheless he recognizes there is danger.

> *But on the flip side, I go through a couple of boxes of 50 pack latex exam gloves per day in my practice and I would venture to say that at least 20% per box are defective either with small pin hole openings or split and tear radically when putting them on. If condoms have as low a quality reliability as the gloves sold to the medical profession then heaven help us all..* [20]

Notes

1. Countries in Central America need to invest more in HIV/AIDS prevention, Revista Hispanoamericana de Salud Pública, Vol. 14, No 6, Dec. 2003.
2. Sex without condom, commonly known as bbfs (Bare Back Full Service)
3. According to the poll taker "It doesn't matter if it is your novia or not. With intent means that the condom did not break, it means she or you just slipped it in."
4. http://www.costaricaticas.com/phpBB2/viewtopic.php?t=4924
5. http://www.costaricaticas.com/phpbb2/viewtopic.php?t=3150
6. http://www.costaricaticas.com/phpbb2/viewtopic.php?t=3150
7. http://www.costaricaticas.com/phpbb2/viewtopic.php?t=3126
8. http://www.costaricaticas.com/phpbb2/viewtopic.php?t=3126
9. http://www.costaricaticas.com/phpbb2/viewtopic.php?t=3126
10. http://www.costaricaticas.com/phpbb2/viewtopic.php?t=3126
11. http://www.costaricaticas.com/phpbb2/viewtopic.php?t=3126
12. http://www.costaricaticas.com/phpbb2/viewtopic.php?t=3126
13. http://www.costaricaticas.com/phpbb2/viewtopic.php?t=3126
14. http://www.costaricaticas.com/phpbb2/viewtopic.php?t=3126
15. http://www.costaricaticas.com/phpbb2/viewtopic.php?t=3126

16. http://www.costaricaticas.com/phpbb2/viewtopic.php?t=3203
17. http://www.costaricaticas.com/phpbb2/viewtopic.php?t=3126
18. http://www.costaricaticas.com/phpbb2/viewtopic.php?t=3203
19. http://www.costaricaticas.com/phpbb2/viewtopic.php?t=3203
20. http://www.costaricaticas.com/phpbb2/viewtopic.php?t=2738

8. *Machismo* and feminism

Sex workers might be very different from their clients in most aspects. Nevertheless, something they both share is resentment toward their own partners. The websites that promote sex tourism provide, for example, some reasons why local women prefer Americans: Latin men, because of their "machismo," have alienated them and this has led them "to look for softer and more enlightened types of masculinity." [1] The majority of sex workers report in our in–depth interviews having being abused physically, mentally and economically by their local partners. Very few of them are married and most of them have children with fathers who have not assumed their paternal responsibility.

María's story is typical [2]. She was born in Turrialba, Costa Rica. She was the sixth of eight siblings, the daughter of a domestic servant and a gardener who fathered five of the eight children and never took care of his own offspring, much less the ones sired by others.

Early on, María remembers that her father would sit her down on his lap and rub her private parts with "something hard." At the time, she had no idea what was going on. The only thing that made her nervous was the father's rapid breathing and what she now describes as a "demented and vigilant look", though she is not sure how she perceived it then. "It was like the panting of a cornered animal," she now says.

However, María recalls that things changed radically when she was 12.

> *Sitting on my father's lap and feeling his member had become part of our relationship. He had told me not to tell my mother or my brothers because what we did was 'private' and the others would feel envious. Sometimes he'd give me money to buy chocolate bars and he would warn me, 'If you talk, you'll have to share the chocolate with everyone."*

This sexual relationship continued for three years. But she never felt strong emotions again. "When my father penetrated me, I did not feel anything, neither pleasure, nor pain, nor disgust or anything. I'd feel like I had left the bed, the room, the house, because I couldn't feel my body. 'You finished?' I'd ask, and if he said yes I'd get dressed and go clean the house as if nothing had happened."

María thinks the relationship with her father helped her in the business. "I have to be honest with you. For me, the fact that I could leave my body or not feel anything when I was having sex has been good for [practicing] prostitution." According to María, it is easier to work as a prostitute when one is detached and can "think of other things." She is convinced that a prostitute's greatest skill is "being able to switch off from what she's doing, and feel pleasure if she wants to." The years with her father "were a training course for this profession," she said.

María does not see herself as a sexual object, or a victim of men. "That's the kind of shit that rich feminists who don't know anything about the poor will say," she commented. "I'm in charge of my body and I sell it.... I don't hand over it for free like many women, in exchange for nothing. I'm better off than the miserable wife who gets a cock shoved up her every night, even if she doesn't want it, and next day she has to be a servant to her husband." She stated that she works at Mas Por Menos supermarket as a front to hide the true profession. "Do you expect me to live from $200 a month? Working 48 hours a week? I do that in an hour at Del Buey."

The relationship between abuse and prostitution is more complex than would appear at first sight. According to our 1993 survey, there is a connection between not using condoms and having suffered punishment or abuse in childhood.[3] María's story suggests that abused girls find ways of "switching off" an unpleasant event while it is happening, which would make it easier to practice prostitution.

Most adults who were abused as children clearly do not practice prostitution or unsafe sex. Many prostitutes feel that their job is not abusive, and that is not really all that different from giving people manicures or a stress–relieving massage. The problem, they say, is the Christian aversion to sex, which considers prostitution not only the oldest profession but also the lowest.

However, the purpose of this work is not to explore why some women choose prostitution, but rather to explain the mutual attraction between American tourists and prostitutes. Although the answer would appear simple –that the men want sex and the women want money– the reality is more complex.

One of the interesting phenomena uncovered by these surveys is the type of men sex workers have as local "*novios*." Most of these men are short, fat and bald. Ana explains that: "Pretty boys are very spoiled and destructive in Costa Rica. In a relationship, I am the only one who is allowed to be attractive. Ugly men are more faithful." This means that these women are not necessarily turned on by male beauty, either in customers or lovers. "Good looks is irrelevant"- says Rita. "It is how men provide me with security what it counts for me; beautiful men are no good for that"- she concludes.

Given this attitude, it is easier for them to find sixty–year–old fat American men attractive and desirable for relationships. "Prostitutes are like cats"- says a taxi driver. "They fall in love with houses and things rather than people." The attraction is not so much for the man but for the type of life he can provide.

American tourists do have an impact on the emotional life of sex workers. They manage to provide the money and respect that these women lack in their local communities. Sex workers are taken to fine restaurants, shops, hotels, casinos, nightclubs, clubs and resorts where they are treated as upper class Latin ladies. This "entrance" to the sphere of the wealthy in Latin America is a passport to the good life and to a higher self–esteem. It affords them the fine food, good wines and champagne, and the fancy clothes otherwise beyond their means. The tourist industry treats them with respect and looks for these women's approval. Businessmen and tour guides covet them for the tourists they bring along

> *My girl knows she has a big fish on the hook. I am there (in CR) every month for work, I pay her well, treat her well, and she may honestly believe that I may bring her out of her current occupation (which she is dang good at, but does not like). Although, her chances of me being the White Knight are slim to none . . . she has a fairy tale of a better life, and I am the star! And when I am there, I treat her like a princess. I don't know how many of you gentlemen have actually seen how most of these women live . . . but it is very sad and depressing. So, when they do get the chance to latch onto a nice gentleman (like most of the gents on this board) they do make the break and show emotion... 4*

It is not difficult to understand why the sex worker becomes hooked to this new standard of living. It empowers them, it makes them gain social approval, it allows them to live the way no one can in thieir local communities. Prostitution also encourages business curiosity and provides training in making money. This is not a trivial pursuit. Most sex workers start selling clothes and jewelry. Through their work they establish business connections and find new ways of making money. Elizabeth, a Colombian sex worker, uses her sex money to import gold chains from Bogotá and sells them to Costa Rican businessmen. Maria imports fabrics from Ecuador and has a small shop in her neighborhood. Teresa sells fine wine from Chile.

This new life can be accessible thanks to either one or many men. If an American tourist is ready to commit and marry, she will have permanent access to the new status. If he is not, she is able to keep her status by having many customers. Whatever the options, the American customer is not her enemy or one who is perceived as exploitative. Sex workers have more resentment against local men than against American tourists. The latter are seen as allies in their struggle to overcome class, gender and educational handicaps.

The problem for these women is that there is very little they can give back for the monger's non–machista treatment. They lack the monger's education, language, sophistication and wealth. The only thing they can provide is sex and some warmth. When the relationship becomes more passionate, bareback sex becomes her final token of appreciation.

Notes

1. www.spanisheyes.com
2. This story is from a study that was previously published in: *Los Traileros y la vida loca* by Jacobo Shifter, The Haworth Hispanic and Latino Studies a division of The Haworth Press, Inc, 1990 pp. 149–153
3. Jacobo Schifter, *Latino Truck Driver Trade. Sex and HIV in Central America,* The Haworth Press, New York: 2001. p.148.
5. http://www.costaricaticas.com/phpbb2/viewtopic.php?t=2738

9. Tradition versus modernity

American men and Costa Rican sex workers are reacting towards gender roles that are either changing too fast, in the case of the former, or not changing fast enough in the case of the latter. Stoller's study in South East Asia viewed the male pursuit of paid sex as a reaction against woman's changing roles:

> *The picture of the client that emerges from these analysis is of men unable to cope with the changing roles of women. They are men seeking a return to a patriarchal system at best, and at worst, are men consumed with (suppressed) hostility towards women.* [1]

Mongers, like Jeff, confessed to feeling despised by American women who are perceived as too emotionally demanding and who are portrayed sometimes as "feminists" and other times as "bitches." Local women as María, on the other hand, feel ill treated by macho men -- from fathers to lovers -- who do not assume their obligations and who tend to be abusive and unfaithful. Our data showed that a history of sexual violence among sex workers fostered emotional detachment. Perhaps divorce, and their former wives' abandonment and rejection, also played a role in the compartmentalization of the American tourist.

Prostitution becomes a theater of sorts for both the sex worker and her client. In this "act," María is being courted as a "lady" and is being lavished with attention, gifts and money, something that was missing from her relationships with local men. In exchange, Jeff gets a loving and nurturing woman who is treated more as a child than an adult woman. Witling describes his relationship with sex workers in terms of education with carrots and sticks.

> *Women are like spoiled Ch*ldren. They are self-focused, insecure and irrational. They demand constant attention, reassurance. And, like Ch*ldren,*

who ceaselessly push limits to see just how much they can get away with from their parents, women relentlessly test men."

1. *Pouting or acting bratty or bitchy when she doesn't get her way, no matter how minor.*
2. *Blaming you when you call her on her behavior.*

The key to dealing with her is also outlined in the article. I've grown much more understanding with time (and 2 previous marriages) but I'm still enough of a hardass to hold her accountable for her actions.

1. (4)- Stand your ground at the outset. At the first inkling of a test, put your foot down, and keep it down. Tell her that you refuse to be tested. Explain to her that if she wants to be with you, then she'll have to knock off the childish behavior.

2. (5)- When all else fails, walk away. This is your ultimate power as a man, and the ultimate "pass" of her tests.

Within no time she is all lovey–dovey again. She knows this ain't my first rodeo and who is in charge. She also knows she is welcome to walk out the door whenever she doesn't like it.

Of course threatening to find another woman doesn't hold much weight because she can find 1000 men for any 1 woman I could get. The funny thing is she is deathly afraid that I MIGHT find a girlfriend. I hope she never realizes how lucky I really am. [2]

Sex workers are not typical women, if we understand this as women who accept a double standard and traditional religious values. Prostitutes are strong and independent women who have chosen greater freedom of movement and action. This freedom of movement is not only geographical since they can journey into men's minds and share an erotic sexuality with them.

Carla, a sex worker from Costa Rica, tells us that she now handles her own money. "As a wife, I never knew what you could do with money, and I could never buy anything for myself because my husband would give me money drop by drop. Now, as a whore, I've got my own money in the bank and I don't rely on some jerk to tell me what to do. When I get fed up with a man I just drop him forever. Not like my mother who had to put up with the drunk she lived with." She says the following about her first paid sexual relationship:

The guy really knew how to please a woman. He gave me oral sex, which I'd never had before, and that was the first time I had an orgasm. But, the real

> *pleasure was getting the $100 bill. Ever since I became a whore, I've learned how important money is, how to save it and how to invest in my business. Before, I had to have sex for free. Now, the guys have to pay.* [3]

Tomasita, from Panama, agrees. "I'm freer as a whore than as a lady. Men think they exploit me, but I'm the one who gets their money and leaves them without a penny. Before, I had to have sex with them if they took me out someplace. Now they have to take me drinking and dining, and on top of that they have to pay." "We dress, eat, and live better than the ladies," says Georgina, "and we have more freedom to pick our men." Alba eats meat every day; before she was a hooker, she says, all she ate was "rice and beans." Emperatriz shows off her clothes; "Now I have fine dresses, not the rags I wore when I was a servant." Luisa thinks she has greater control over her sexuality; "I get my orgasm with whichever customer I want. If there's one I don't like, I wait until the next. I can tell him what I want and when. With my boyfriend, I had to lie there looking at the ceiling until he came." But with the first American client, she felt different.

The American tourist is willing to play this role of temporary and substitute father and lover. In exchange for such performance, he gets the traditional feminine performance.

Some of the stereotypes about sexual roles are questioned by the sex tourism industry. Prostitution is usually described as an institution that objectifies and uses women. Men are thought to be more physical and with a greater tendency to have sex without an emotional commitment. Women, on the other hand, are taught to engage in sex only in the context of a loving relationship.

This reality is contradicted by monger culture. American tourists are adamant about their desire to become loving and share feelings. Eljefe, for example, is aware of the gender dichotomy but nevertheless thinks that mongers are not typical males and that they embrace femininity:

> *The GFE supposes that emotional attachment, even if for a decidedly short period. So, by extension, those pursuing the GFE are embracing, perhaps, feminine sexual connections (I assume all are in this for the sex, no?). Yet everybody (well, almost) needs to beaccepted, desired, loved. Oriental philosophy (or which I am no scholar) describes this phenomenon, called the yin and the yang.* [4]

Astroglide states that the Girlfriend Fantasy Experience (GFE) is synonymous with emotional involvement. "If you want to get off in 15 minutes and throw them out you are not a GFE guy. If you insist in spending the full hour with them, and then beg them to stay longer, you are a GFE guy. If, when they are finished, you send them back alone, you are not a GFE guy. But if you insist on walking them back . . . or even asking them out again . . . You are looking for a GFE. If you want to spend time with them, get in their head, take them out of the gulch and maybe even spend money on them, you are looking for a GFE."[5] In their wish for emotional relationships, mongers think they are different from those "Tico bangers who want to get their rocks off in the shortest time possible and leave' em. They really grow up thinking sex is a 15 minute experience."[6]

Mongers spend time in buying perfumes, flowers and chocolates. They also use scents and candles to enliven the sexual relationship. They seem to be the ones responsible for seducing cold and materialistic women, who only want to use and exploit them. Astroglide provides the following advice on love–making: "Lesson #1: Teach them how to have sex your way. Spend time with them. Play the Magic CD. Light the candles. Lesson #2: Control the environment. Never let them watch TV. YOU set the mood and the atmosphere. That's why the candles and the CD are great ideas. It allows you to create a romantic mood, instead of just a banging and leave' em experience."[7]

Despite their lack of command of the Spanish language, they want to talk and share their emotions and thoughts with others. They want the women to be in touch with their feelings and hidden thoughts. Astroglide summarizes in the next rules of his love–making proposal: "Lesson #3: Get inside their heads. Show them that you care. Ask them about their families and the K*ds. Let them tell you about their hijos. Let them relax. Let them see you as a real person, and you must see them as the same. Show them respect and treat them like little princesses. They will respond in kind."[8]

Contrary to the expectation that men only think of sex, some mongers feel so emotional that they forego sex for cuddling and touching since they only want to feel close to a woman: "I do like sex –says Coyote– but recently, I have had nights where I was even with a girl and just relaxed with no sex."[9]

They also share their feelings with other men. Mongers repeatedly state that one of the reasons they love Costa Rica is because they can be with other fellow mongers and enjoy their company. A monger admitted one of the perks of a Costa Rican vacation was to meet other men: " One big reason is the guys I've met and become friends with through CRT."[10] They establish friendships that last for many years and they miss each other when one monger disappears from the Forums: "On June 23rd, after 789 posts, CostaKid seemed to fall off the face of the earth. At least that is the last post I could find. I realize that people come and go here, and maybe they have to disappear with no warning . . . but that seems odd to me. Maybe I will find him on the beach at Jaco with a long beard, an old t–shirt and a shit eating grin on his face. Are there others that have gone into the ether without a trace?"[11]

Mongers seem to feminize themselves during their Costa Rican holiday, which provides an opportunity to escape from traditional American life and masculinity. Shields[12], Rojek[13] and Ryan[14] have alluded to medieval periods of disorder when discussing holidays. During such time breaks, settled order was set aside, the jester became king and hierarchies were challenged, albeit within a temporary framework." The same is enacted in modern times as sex tourists let themselves be what they do not allow themselves to be at home.

This disorder might be thought as rather positive since it is an opportunity to explore alternative behaviors and friendships with both men and women. Nevertheless, it might become rather troublesome for HIV prevention since passivity, willingness to please others and emotionality might lead to taking risks.

Notes

1. A. Stoler, "Educating Desire in Colonial SouthEast Asia: Foucault, Freud ad imperial sexualities," in L. Manderson and Jolly (eds) *Sites of Desire, Economics of Pleasure: Sexualities in Asia and the Pacific,* Chicago: University of Chicago Press, 1997, p.154.
2. http://www.costaricaticas.com/phpbb2/viewtopic.php?t=3729
3. http://www.costaricaticas.com/phpbb2/viewtopic.php?t=3729
4. http://www.costaricaticas.com/phpbb2/viewtopic.php?t=82&postdays=0&postorder=asc&highlight=sending+money&start=30
5. http://www.costaricaticas.com/phpbb2/viewtopic.php?t=82&highlight=sending+money
6. http://www.costaricaticas.com/phpbb2/viewtopic.php?t=82&highlight=sending+money
7. http://www.costaricaticas.com/phpbb2/viewtopic.php?t=82&highlight=sending+money
8. http://www.costaricaticas.com/phpbb2/viewtopic.php?t=82&highlight=sending+money
9. http://www.costaricaticas.com/phpbb2/viewtopic.php?t=3969
10. http://www.costaricaticas.com/phpbb2/viewtopic.php?t=3969
11. http://www.costaricaticas.com/phpbb2/viewtopic.php?t=4191
12. R. Shields, Places on the Margin: Alternative Geographies of Modernity, London: Routledge, 1991.
13. C. Rojek, *Ways of Escape: Modern Transformations in Leisure and Travel,* London: MacMillan, 1993.
14. C. Ryan, *The Tourist Experience: A New Introduction, London:* Cassel, 1997.

10. Liminal

Chris Ryan and C. Michael Hall portray "Mongers" and sex workers as "liminal" creatures.[1] This means –despite the persecution being heavier on the women– that they share an identity of illegality and transgression.

> *The act of sex tourism can therefore be explained as an interaction between two sets of liminal people –but with a difference. The one, the tourist, is enacting a socially sanctioned and economically empowered marginality, while the second, the prostitute, is stigmatized as a whore, a woman of the night, a scarlet woman.*[2]

Sex work, whether legal or not, is socially looked down upon in Western societies and prostitution has an old historically negative connotation. María cannot admit openly what her real profession is. She has to listen to her priest's sermons that condemn "loose" women and who preach that prostitution is the worst calamity the country suffers from. Her two children curse other children with the worst offense that can be uttered in Spanish: "Hijodeputa" (Sonofabitch). If one of the former Costa Rican lovers, and fathers of her children, find out she is working at Del Buey, they can take her to court and take away her custody over them.

Both the prostitute and her client are forced to live hidden sexual lives outside the law.

American mongers admit feeling discrimination, misunderstanding and the need to hide their sexual preferences. Jsmythe23, for example, responds to the Detroit Post without having read the article on prostitution, assuming it will be prejudiced. He believes the Detroit paper, ABC, has the right to write on Costa Rican prostitution. Nevertheless, he is sure the article will be "cheap and salacious." Jsmythe23 anticipates that the journalist will ignore the fact that prostitution is legal in Costa Rica and that no minors are allowed inside the hotels that cater to sex tourists. "ID's are required at the door"- he states. He also thinks that the paper will neglect the fact that many young women in Costa Rica pay their university studies thanks to prostitution. They would not acknowledge, "the sex industry is not managed by pimps as it is the case in the States." America is so "puritanical," he added, that the Mafia is the one who rules prostitution and it is the one that forces sex workers into consuming drugs. "This is not the case in this Central American country, but the paper will not admit it." –He wrote. "They also will not write that prostitution is a common practice in the civilized world. Their goal will be to shock the audience and to show mongers as perverts and criminals." He hypothetically posed a question regarding the issue: "What is that you want?. For Costa–Rica to apply the same ineffective and harmful laws that the U.S. has regarding prostitution so that women can get forced out of the safety of secure nightclubs and hotels and work on the street getting beat–up, exploited by pimps, harassed by police etc?" [3]

Since mongers feel themselves misunderstood and persecuted, they tend to establish their own dialects, geographical spaces, sexual behavior and meeting places. They share the fears of other persecuted groups. They must be wary of strangers who might turn them in, of hidden cameras in the nightclubs and hotels, and of their own non–monger friends. They believe the journalists are to "out" them, only to increase their newspaper's ratings. Given this situation, Jsmythe23 proposes the following rules of conduct:

1. *Be careful who you meet down there. NEVER reveal your true identity.*
2. *Be careful who PM's you on this board. If it is a newbie, somebody you have never met personally, do NOT reveal your true identity.*
3. *If a user here gets pushy and attempts to find out who you are, report them to the Admins.*
4. *Always exit any house of prostitution with a wary eye. If you see a camera crew . . . RUN. Do not look back. They can't ID you from behind.*
5. *Never . . . EVER go with an underage prostitute. Make her show ID. If she can't . . . leave her alone. Always assume that maybe SHE has a hidden camera. Be careful even just TALKING to a minor in public.*
6. *Be careful who you talk to about this hobby of ours. If you don't know them and trust them . . . decir nada!*
7. *Never post anything in this board or any other message board that could help somebody easily ID you.*

I hate to be this paranoid . . . but you HAVE to be. Trust me on this, mi amigos. This is not going away. Remember the old line from Candid Camera? One day, when you least expect it . . . SMILE . . . you're on Candid Camera." In an instant, your life can be exposed, and if you are in a sensitive situation . . . ruined. [4]

It is no secret that groups that are discriminated against tend to alleviate their burden by many different means. The tourist sex industry is filled with adrenaline hikes such as gambling, drugs and sex. Mongers admit that Costa Rica has become a sort of "crack cocaine" that is hard to control. Don Gordo, for example, has made 59 trips to Costa Rica during the last decade; others have come more than 20 times. As Prolijo indicates bellow this means spending money, time and energy on women, alcohol and gambling. Once the high is felt, it is hard to stop.

> *It's definitely an addiction. Whether it is like drug abuse depends on the individual. Like drug abuse, the "chica fix" can detract from our drive to deal with "relationship" issues in a more complete and long–term way. It can act as a means to or at least a substitute for many of the things one normally gets from more traditional relationships, beginning with sex but also including, companionship, ego gratification or whatever. If going to CR for short term "fixes" take away from ones effort or drive to seek out more fulfilling relationships (or ones with long term potential), it could be a sign of "drug" abuse. .* [5]

Sex seems to be the major high for mongers:

> *We go to CR because we love to phuck, to fulfill our lust and fantasies– it's a quick–fix, an escape from our reality, the bitchy–cold wife/GF or loneliness and everything else at home, the rush of leading a double life, with women that are so hot and sweet. And we can phuck all we want without all the complications and crap we'd normally have to put up with. What guy in here hasn't fantasized about phucking hot young women since puberty, and after many rejections, failed relationships, marriages, whatever, found CR and finally able to "catch–up" and make it come true.* [6]

Women and sex are not the only monger's "highs." Hotel Del Buey and the rest of the nightclubs also include casinos where many of the customers gamble all night. After all, both sex and games offer random and unexpected rewards. You can choose the most beautiful girl in the hotel and this is no guarantee that the sex will be great. The loving woman in the lobby can become detached and cold in the bedroom. Some fake their orgasms and others have real orgasms. Sometimes it is the women who want more sex and do not charge extra for it. Both casinos and the bedrooms provide similar random pleasures and risks: It is quite easy to become addicted to both.

> *That last paragraph reminds me of one morning about a year ago at about 7 am in San José I was walking from the Morazan to the Colonial to have breakfast.*

I saw a guy who looked obviously like a gringo and looked to be in bad shape, like something bad had happened to him. My first intuition was that he was suffering from a hangover. I asked him if he was OK –he said no and that he was "out of control." I said, "you mean out of control about sex." (I was thinking about myself and the only thing I could imagining myself being out of control about in CR)
He laughed bitterly and said, "hell no, I wish it was sex –I am out of control with my gambling. Now I have to go home to my wife." I felt very badly for the guy and offered to buy him breakfast and talk to him but he said he had to go home.[7]

Sex worker themselves are addicted. They also expect to win the Big Prize either in gambling or in sex. Rosaura admits, “Most of my money is wasted in gambling.” Lourdes, another sex worker, spends 50,000 colones a night in poker. José, a security guard at the Casino Del Buey believes sex workers gamble half of their earnings.

If is not in gambling, the women are hooked to cocaine, alcohol or shopping.

Some sex workers owe street vendors and/or salesmen more than a month’s income. This is mostly due to the fact that they have to constantly reinvent themselves through new clothing, jewelry and perfumes.

María admitted that “there is something out of control in our lives.” Being “hooked” makes them feel powerless. Lupe, a sex worker, feelt she could not control her unsafe sexual behavior because “I cannot stop my gambling habits.” Miriam feelt helpless with regard to alcohol; “I cannot stop drinking after my 10th drink. I don’t remember what I do when I am drunk.”

Alcohol consumption is a major problem for sex workers. Almost two thirds of the 2000 survey drank alcohol, 30% did it more than once a week and 10% drank everyday. Of the sample, 38% has done other drugs and 13% consumed mainly marihuana and cocaine. (Tables 8–9)

Among drug users, cocaine seemed to hold a larger attraction than marijuana. (Table 10) Those who have consumed the drug and those who consume it were almost the same. In the case of marijuana, those who have consumed it (26%) were larger as a group than those who were consuming it (18%). On the other hand, according to the survey, crack consumption was reduced to zero among drug users (11% have consumed it and 0 were consuming it.) Nevertheless, our other sources of information revealed that this was not the case. Sex workers who lived mostly off alcohol sales were using crack cocaine to lessen alcohol intoxication so they could be able to sell more drinks to themselves and their clients.

Of the sex workers who consumed drugs, 54% did so every day. Sex workers were also mixing more alcohol and sex (49%) than drugs and sex (10%). The data indicated that alcohol is the drug most used to have sex.

From the information we gathered in our ethnographic observations, in–depth interviews and focus groups, we sense that the problem of alcohol consumption is increasing and more serious than the 2000 survey revealed. Those sex workers who work in nightclubs make their salaries more from the sale of alcohol than sex.

These women have two sources of income: nude dancing and a percentage of the sales from alcohol to clients. Puro Placer Night–Club, for example, has an admittance fee of approximately $12. The client only gets one drink and is expected to consume much more. The sex workers get 20% per drink served both to her and her client. Champagne is the drink most ordered by the sex workers and each drink is approximately $7. A private dance to the customer is $10 and this goes mostly to the sex worker. If the client wants a private booth to get nude dancing and some petting, masturbation or oral sex he must order a bottle of champagne, which costs $200. In the Elite Night Club the minimum consumption fee is $15. The champagne bottle needed to get a private booth is $270.

This system is called "*fichaje*," ("chip," in Spanish.) The waiters keep the number of "chips" the sex worker is making throughout the evening and her salary is determined accordingly. Therefore, it is implicit that the client and the sex worker should drink as much as possible. The client also pays those drinks served to the women.

From our focus group we learned that a sex worker could order as many as 40 drinks per night. They indicated that the number of drinks needed to get intoxicated was 19. They admitted that after this number they lost control over their behavior and sexual practice. Some women in our focus groups–discussions admitted to having forgotten to use condoms when intoxicated and usually did not recall what they did with their clients. Others reported that clients became violent and more aggressive when they were aware that the sex worker was drunk.

An average client can spend almost $300 in one evening and sex workers can make from $500 to $1500 per month just on alcohol sales. If the client wants to have sex outside of the premises he must pay another $200 to the bar owners plus the same amount to the sex worker.

Some waiters help the sex workers by mixing soda with the champagne and reducing in this manner the amount of alcohol. Nevertheless, this is not possible when the client orders a bottle. Clients want the sex workers to drink since this allows them to have more control over them and for this reason they usually check the drinks to see if they have not been altered. When this occurs the attempts to reduce alcohol consumption by the waiters fail. One of the alternatives for the sex workers is to smoke cocaine, which reduces intoxication. We observed many sex workers using cocaine in the bathrooms or doing it prior to entering into the bars.

In 2000, 71% of sex workers responded having problems in using condoms when mixing alcohol and sex. This pattern can be due to the increasing participation of sex workers in the "fichaje" system. As profits are shifting from prostitution to alcohol sales, sex workers are increasingly more vulnerable to intoxication and unsafe sex. Despite the prevention efforts carried by the government and NGO's, alcohol intoxication is becoming a serious obstacle to safer sex.

From the in–depth interviews we learned that the problem for sex workers when intoxicated is aggravated by the client's refusal to use condoms. As they also get intoxicated, the demand to not use condoms increases.

Alcohol consumption seems to be the major factor of risk for unsafe sex both for the sex worker and her client. There is also a strong link with cocaine consumption. From our ethnographic observation we learned that sex workers use crack cocaine to lessen intoxication and to allow them to consume more drinks. This increasing need for cocaine forces them to spend more money on this drug and, accordingly, increase the need for more income from alcohol sales. This is a vicious cycle that leads them to make clients drink more and expose themselves to more pressures for having unsafe sex.

Another phenomenon that was concealed by the interviewees in the 2000 survey is that crack and cocaine use has increased considerably over the last few years. Sex workers in Costa Rica fill the discussion forums with commentaries about the high levels of crack consumption. Charles illustrates in a newsgroup a particular situation with a sex worker in Costa Rica who ran from the hotel room before the sexual act had concluded. To this Goetz responds

> *Barring any strange occurrence between the two of you during the exercise, if she abruptly stopped during the middle of the hump and got pissed either she was not planning on really doing the two hours, at least not actively or had something else going on. The fact that she seemed to have a personality change and forgot about the money leads me to believe she was on something. I have had a lot of experience with girls on coke and crack in my old strip club days and I promise you they can go night and day in a heartbeat without any obvious signs of use. They will go psychotically paranoid in a flash, have 180 degree mood swings and be completely irrational...* [8]

Charles agrees with him and believes half of the women are on coke: "I have noticed this, can recognize "jonesing" demeanors, and would not be surprised if about half of them are on coke. Very sad considering how destructive that stuff is."[9]

Monger culture is an alcohol culture. Not only is sex tourism an escapade from daily work and obligations, which provides an excuse for people to drink more than usual, but provides a space that allows men to express their feelings. The means to do this in Western culture is usually through intoxication. Since sharing feelings is what they do in Costa Rica, no wonder then they need so much alcohol.

The discussion forums are filled with stories of drunken Americans at the bars. Gringotim, for example, describes the alcohol consumption of a 22 year old Canadian tourist at La Cantina, the bar at the hotel Irazú: "This k*d, in an hour and 15 minutes, drank two Imperials, two shots of Tequila, two Ron Centenarios Y Cokes, and some Guaro. I'm thinking "this k*d is out of control!." Sure enough, he puts his hand to his mouth as if to burp, then proceeds to puke right on the bar! It was disgusting! [10]

DEAR_JOHN reveals that a guy from Nevada was doing cocaine and talking about having sex with children. [11] Tunaman reports on the "generic drunk" American who makes a fool of himself and whom sex workers run away from. "I have only witnessed the generic drunk gringo assholes. One time, this drunk sits next to me at the bar in the BM. He tries to talk with some chicas in his version of Spanish, which is just adding an "O" at the end of any English word. I can tell these girls don't even want to deal with his drunken ass for any amount of $$$. ...Usually the drunks that expect Latinas to kiss his ass are a little weary of going someplace where the locals hang out." [12]

Prolijo shares a typical story:

> *I was with VB when the surfer dude was doing his thing. First he lifted his arms as if to stretch, but I think he was just trying to show off his muscles. The bar was very crowded at the time. So next he proceeded to swing his elbows around violently knocking people out of the way saying "time to make some room around here" as if he thought it was the funniest thing anyone ever said or did. VB, who had been sitting with me at the bar, got pushed aside. VB looked like he was ready to stand his ground and take a swing at the guy. But I suggested it was time for us to circulate anyway. I'm glad I talked VB out of it. That guy may have been drunk but he was sure damn BIG.* [13]

It is hard to tell at this point how much alcohol dependency there is among American sex tourists. But the anecdotal evidence suggests it is a major concern and a strong factor in predicting unsafe sex. Tourists say that there is little to do in San José but drink. The majority brings their own booze with them. Most, since they are on holidays, probably drink more often than in the United States. The fact is that most people who work in the sex industry report that most Americans are drunk for the duration of their trips. The Blue Marylin, the small bar at Hotel Del Buey, makes a profit of more than $10,000 a month, according to the manager.

Alcohol intoxication is one of the major factors for unsafe sex among sex workers and it is likely to be also for their clients.

Another addiction among American tourists is to Viagra, CIALIS and Levitra. According to the Survey at costaricaticas.com, Viagra, called "Vitamin V" is by far the most popular among sex tourists. [14] These drugs allow middle–aged men to have full erections for longer periods of time. Goetz, for instance, is totally convinced that Levitra is "the hands down winner." According to him, its effects can last for days. He uses it because it "restores my abilities to my 18 year old level." He knows that many mongers share this since "Most of us have led similar lifestyles and after a certain level of age and abuse we need a little help. It has nothing to do with desire, more to do with prolonged alcohol consumption, high triglycerides, obesity, lack of exercise, Propecia, borderline diabetes, smoking, poor diet, and all the other pleasurable things that mongers do. If you are over 40 and do any of the above you will feel the need sooner than later." [15]

One thing is to get a "little help from your friends" and another is to use these drugs as candy. Administrator 3 warns that Viagra and the other sex–enhancing drugs "was first marketed as a heart attack pill that dilates arteries and increases blood flow to the heart. It wasn't a big seller until patients mentioned a raging hard–on as a side effect. Phizer repositioned the drug as a sexual–enhancement pill and the rest is history." The drug works, he says, but "overdosing" (taking more than the daily prescribed amount) is a threat. A possible outcome is the "gringo dropping dead at the El Duende because of overdosing." He thinks this American sex tourist "drank a whole bottle of Viagra in two days!" [16]

Viagra is for people who have problems getting erections because of diabetes, old age or other illnesses. It is not a drug prescribed for having sex with several prostitutes in a single day or for having sex for five hours in a row. Nevertheless, this is the main reason the drug is taken and tourists increase the dosage to be able to experience sex again as in their younger days. A twenty–six year old monger, for example, admits " In 48 hours I had around 12 pops with Cialis." He writes that he came to Costa Rica only for a weekend and "The day before the trip I went to the gym and got a really hard workout and got 3 d–bols from a friend just to increase my tetosteronne [sic] levels and sex drive." Once in Costa Rica, "I was like a maniac the first night, then leveled off." He advices other mongers that when taking Cialis is better "no masturbation 24 hours prior to the trip since it will keep you erect as long as you take it." The only problem with the drug for him is that "just eventually run outa juice. But, as long as you have juice on Cialis, you can really just keep going and going, like the energizer bunny, no shit, just remember to change condoms in between loads." [17]

Another young monger who is 30 years old, is intrigued about what to do:

"I will be in Costa Rica on Saturday night for one week. Today is Wednesday and I have roughly four days before the fun begins. I need advice on masturbating prior to my trip. Should I withhold from masturbating for the next four days so that I am really horny and build up my reserves or should I continue masturbating twice a day so my body will be ready for the excitement when I am down there."[18]

It becomes evident that tourists do self–prescribe and that the high consumption of sex–enhancing drugs is mainly for keeping up with the active monger life in Costa Rica, something that looks dangerous to their health.

> *Gentlemen,*
>
> *Just a heads up on Viagra use . . . I read on one or more posts about people popping Viagra more than once a day and wanted to give a warning about such use. I myself was popping one every 6–8 hours for a time span of 4 days and found out later how utterly stupid and dangerous that was and wanted to share some info.*
>
> *Here's what I want to let everyone know . . . The erection effects of the pill lasts about 4 hours on average. HOWEVER, you should NOT take more than 1 pill in a 24 hour period. Although the erection effects last only 4 hours, the compound is in your system for 24 hours and taking more than one in a 24 hour period puts you at risk of bottoming out your blood pressure. Risks of disorientation, dizziness, severe headache, passing out (and hurting yourself in the process) are REAL when over medicating. Yes, even death may happen to someone with pre–existing medical conditions to complicate this effect. Just thought everyone should be educated on this risk for future precautions...*[19]

This is a topic that merits more research. Nevertheless, the post bellow indicates there are other health threats caused by sex–enhancing drugs that we might not be even aware of. DBCocker writes this weird story in capital letters to call everyone's attention.

> *IT SEEMS HE GOT A LITTLE INTOXICATED ON THE FLIGHT TO CR AND WAS FEELING NO PAIN SO ON ARRIVAL HE GOES STRIGHT TO HOTEL CHECKS IN THEN TO THE DB TO PICK UP A CHICIA. BACK TO HOTEL HE'S GOT HER IN BED WITH HER LEGS OVER HER HEAD REALLY LAYING THE WOOD TO HER I MEAN PHUCKING HER HARD; REMEMBER HE'S TWO SHEETS TO WIND FROM THE FLIGHT DOWN; WELL IT SEEMS HE OVER STROKED AND JAMMED HIS STIFFY INTO HER TAINT SO HARD IT FOLDED HIS C*ck IN HALF CAUSING EXCRUCIATING PAIN FOR BOTH HE AND HIS CHICA . WHEN HE LOOKED DOWN AT HIS WILLY HE SAW THAT IT WAS BENT IN HALF BUT*

WHEN HE REACH DOWN TO STRAIGHTEN IT OUT BLOOD SQUIRTED ALL OVER THE CHICA, THE BED AND THE FLOOR.[20]

Notes

1. Chris Ryan and C. Michael Hall, *Sex Tourism. Marginal People and Liminalities.* Routledge, London and New York, 2001, p.1.
2. Chris Ryan and C. Michael Hall, *Sex Tourism. Marginal People and Liminalities.* Routledge, London and New York, 2001, p.1.
3. http://www.costaricaticas.com/phpbb2/viewtopic.php?t=2173
4. http://www.costaricaticas.com/phpbb2/viewtopic.php?t=2173
5. http://www.costaricaticas.com/phpbb2/viewtopic.php?t=3969
6. http://www.costaricaticas.com/phpbb2/viewtopic.php?t=3969
7. http://www.costaricaticas.com/phpbb2/viewtopic.php?t=3969
8. http://www.costaricaticas.com/phpbb2/viewtopic.php?t=3149
9. http://www.costaricaticas.com/phpbb2/viewtopic.php?t=3149
10. http://www.costaricaticas.com/phpbb2/viewtopic.php?t=2424
11. http://www.costaricaticas.com/phpbb2/viewtopic.php?t=2424
12. http://www.costaricaticas.com/phpbb2/viewtopic.php?t=2424
13. http://www.costaricaticas.com/phpbb2/viewtopic.php?t=2424
14. http://www.costaricaticas.com/phpbb2/viewtopic.php?t=1659
15. http://www.costaricaticas.com/phpbb2/viewtopic.php?t=1659
16. http://www.costaricaticas.com/phpbb2/viewtopic.php?t=2857
17. http://www.costaricaticas.com/phpbb2/viewtopic.php?t=476
18. http://www.costaricaticas.com/phpbb2/viewtopic.php?t=476
19. http://www.costaricaticas.com/phpBB2/viewtopic.php?t=4413
20. http://www.costaricaticas.com/phpbb2/viewtopic.php?t=4066

11. Latin women versus American women

The forum participants are pretty open about the reasons why they look for paid sex. Some don't feel attractive enough to court young and beautiful women. Sixteen percent admitted that one of the reasons for mongering is "You are too hopelessly ugly to get laid at home (not like Circus who can't get laid period)." The majority, are hostile toward American women, who they perceive as aggressive, rude and not "feminine." In a poll taken at CostaRicas.Ticas.com, mongers want to know why they come to Costa Rica. Forty percent responded that they do it because "You hate *gringas* and love *latinas* and only work at home to make money to go to Costa Rica and live." [1]

Why do they hate American women? LVSeve has been married three times; what he dislikes of them is "having to pay for alimony." [2] PacoLoco advises everyone in the sex forums not to marry American women; his reasons are different from LVSteve's. He hates "The bandsaw whine of anger, anger, anger that makes American women an international horror. It's there. It's real." [3] Dman agrees with him. He is still married but if he had to do it again "I would never ever marry again a Gringa." [4]

CapoD2T detests American women of his age because in spite of being "well on the other side of their best day, demand expensive dinners and wining and dining and don't see themselves as "dilapidated and with wrinkled faces" [5] Goal accuses American women of fearing life: "The most disturbing issue about gringas is they are afraid of EVERYTHING, too much American television I suppose." Ablissman is convinced that "I WILL NEVER AGAIN HAVE SEX WITH A WOMAN WHO SPEAKS ENGLISH AS A FIRST LANGUAGE!!!!" He thinks that for American women "EVERYTHING is a political issue. Perhaps there are reasons that have caused this . . . BUT I DO NOT HAVE TO BE A VICTIM OF IT!!!" [6] Pacatelo not only agrees but also contributes to the thread.

For him, American women are undesirable because of their attitude: "The women in the states have to be the least desirable on the planet, and it is the attitude pure and simple." [7] Duardo admits that there might be some few exceptions to the rule but that most American women when they get older they leave no room for discussions or for compromise: "Gringas are definitely on the low side of my opinion level.. Hate to sound so harsh and I dont mean it towards everyone one of them as there are some quality ladies around. But they are so, few and far between and as they have grown older and jaded it has become apparent we can not win.. SO Dont feel so bad you are in great company, as I think the large portion of single guys on this board who have visited and experienced Latin America, South America and countries similar feel just like you..."[8] Bombero, finally, summarizes what he dislikes about gringas and it is not pretty: he sees them as conniving, hypocritical and selfish: "I WILL NEVER HAVE SEX WITH A WOMAN WHO'S RAISED UP IN THE U.S. PERIOD!!!! American woman are conniving, selfish, manipulating, dirty bitches." [9]

This hostility is played on Costa Rican ground when the American female tourist meets the American male tourist. Let's see what happens when a monger finds in Costa Rica a woman his age and she reproaches him for dating a girl who might be his daughter:

> *True story Last trip Me & my Novia were simply walking down Avenida Central looking for sunglasses.. She is holding my arm and we are strolling. OK now she is 19 going on 20 but real TINY . . . . Gringa Bitch about 45–50 comes out of the store as we are window shopping Stares right through me with vengeful eyes and says "I CERTAINLY HOPE THAT IS YOUR DAUGHTER" . . . . Well my Novia Smiled, I smiled then I looked directly back at her and said Next time I certainly hope you mind our own PHUCKING BUSINESS."..*
> *They just can't handle the fact THEY Get old and there isn't a god dam thing they can do about it . . . . Think about it we are 30, 40 50 or older plus and we can still "DATE" if we choose even in the States women that are more than half our age . . . Who the PHUCK wants some dilapidated grapefruit, wrinkled 40 plus miserable Phucking gringa . . . Hmm think I've had enough of the Gringas?*[10]

Some would argue that mongers are reacting against the advancements made by women in the States during the last decades. Nevertheless, it is not so simple. Mongers admit to being also very attracted toward Latin culture, a culture they identify with warmth and a more natural attitude toward flirting and physical attraction.

> *I was driving downtown one day and stopped at a red light at an intersection when an incredibly beautiful Tica started crossing the street. She*

was enjoying all the looks of adoration and howls from onlookers when the light suddenly changed. Everyone remained motionless, hypnotized and with their jaw hanging down (at least mine certainly was!) in dumbstruck tribute and reverence . . . There was a moment of respectful awe and silence. No one moved to cross the intersection until she was almost gone –all four lanes were stopped in every direction for blocks, people in the back were honking angrily and we had to wait until the light changed again before we could cross! It was incredibly funny and I loved it. The women who were standing nearby watching just screamed with laughter, calling us "Canes" (from Canis familiaris) in Spanish, which means "dogs"! Things like that happen all the time in Costa Rica and are to me what make it a welcome change from the boring and smug attitude of many women in the U.S. This is also one of the big reasons why tens of thousands of American men go to Latin America every year, believe it or not! [11]

O'Connell Davidson traces similar attitudes of British sex tourists in Thailand. [12] This implies that the market for these "exotic–erotic" trips is for men that are unable to cope with the self–confident of the West, and there is evidence for such a thesis. Seabrok describes this situation thus:

Westerners think that sex is the ultimate human experience. The young women and men of Bangkok know better. Because these farangs are so lonely, because they are such isolated individuals, they imagine that it is through sex that human beings come closer to one another. They think they see the profoundest communication in what is the loneliest experience in the world. They think like this because they are so far away from each other, they have to reach across the empty spaces of their separateness before they touch another human being. [13]

On the contrary, Latin women are perceived as feminine, submissive, warm and willing to please men. Americans are also aware that age–asymmetrical relationships are more common in Latin America. This means that in Costa Rica it is more common that older males marry younger women than in the United States. A middle–aged strolling around with a young woman does not call people's attention as it would in the United States.

Costa Rican women generally prefer somewhat older men and it is very common to see a beautiful 20–year–old girl with a 40+ year–old man. I heard an American woman say to one of these girls once, "Young lady, why don't you find a boyfriend of your own age!? Why do you go around with a man old enough to be your father? An American woman would never do something like that." (The American woman thought the girl would think just like an American) The girl responded, "Why don't you mind your own business"? What has age got to do with it? And look at you! Why would any man your age be interested in someone that looks like you? You're just resentful and jealous because no one even looks at you anymore." [14]

Mongers also have erroneous beliefs about what makes Latin culture different. They think people are warmer and more flirtatious because there is no gender consciousness and no sex liberation movements.

> *Women's liberation, the feminist movement, and gay rights don't even exist, and the same goes for most of the rest of Latin America except that it is even more so in countries like Brazil (yes I know there are a lot of gays in Brazil, temporarily anyway). If you're against this kind of thinking, you should forget about living in Latin America altogether because you'll run into a real brick wall as far as attempting to confront or change those customs is concerned and you will turn many of the Ticos against you.* [15]

Mongers tend to confuse the political with the cultural. The fact is that the women's movement in Costa Rica was born in the 1920's and there are as many gay establishments in San José as there are in Miami or in Washington D.C.

Some mongers are aware that what they get in Costa Rica is not due to political naiveté, lack of gender consciousness or "primitive" gender relations, but also a performance of what Americans think Latin women should behave. One of the experts in this field, the Administrator of the most popular website on Costa Rican sexual tourism, for example, explains how the "ideal hooker" should act:

> *Here is what I think it takes to be a good hooker in CR.*
>
> 1. *Provide excellent customer service, e.g. smile, be friendly, work hard to satisfy a guy, don't be a clock watcher, provide excellent value for the money.*
> 2. *Dress nicely, wear clean clothes, don't dress like too much of a slut but still dress sexy. Provide an appearance that a guy wants to be seen with.*
> 3. *Be dependable; if you accept a date for a certain time be on time.*
> 4. *Work smart – if you can develop a steady long term customer that pays well then take care of that guy.*
> 5. *Learn as much English as possible to increase your marketability.*
> 6. *Try to remember this is only a way to make some good money; be friendly and remain a human being but remember these guys are basically there just to have sex and affection for relatively short times with you.*
> 7. *Watch some really good porn videos and study how to provide super excellent bj's. No need to swallow that stuff since swallowing is basically an extra for guys.*
> 8. *Take a shower before and after every sex episode; encourage your john to*

take a shower also before sex.

9. *Ask him for an e–mail address if he was good to you; then e–mail him an occasional affectionate message and if he answers then stay at it. It will drive him crazy with anticipation and might make him think you care about him.*
10. *If you have been with a guy and the money was good then be very affectionate with him in public – especially around other guys. Remember that nearly all men are extremely insecure and have very fragile egos. Stroke his arm and leg and remember to lean your breasts on him every chance you have.*
11. *When you are walking in front of men remember to gently sway your hips and ass – not too much but just enough to get them thinking you know your way around the bedroom.*
12. *Price competitively but do not underprice your time and skills. Think gringo pricing and tell them it will be $89 –and smile some of the gringos will think they are getting a bargain and all will laugh.*
13. *Stand and walk alone – it makes it easier for a guy to approach you.*
14. *Don't grope guys walking through the gauntlet –it makes you appear desperate.*
15. *Try bringing a "serious" book to the DB and order a drink and pretend to read the book – make sure the book is in English. Something by Kerouac or some hip writer would be great. Guys will think you are both intelligent and hip.*
16. *Establish eye contact and flirt with your eyes if you see some guy looking at you; pretend you are really a bit shy.*
17. *If he asks you out for dinner –accept the offer if you have been with him before but don't charge for your time for the dinner. Do not order the most expensive things on the menu the first time. Save the expensive choices for later dinners with him.*
18. *If he offers to take you shopping, at first say no and blush. He will almost certainly ask a second time and then you should pretend to be embarrassed and accept the shopping offer. Pick out sothing inexpensive that he can buy you the first time you go shopping – save the expensive stuff for later shopping trips.*
19. *Tell him you are only doing this kind of work to support your mother who is out of work and your brother who is in a wheel chair and unable to work.*
20. *Constantly tell the guy he is handsome and nice; much nicer than the local men or other gringos.*

Note: I am available for career counseling for any DB working girls!" [16]

Do mongers treat Latin sex workers with the same consideration?

The answer is not a positive one. Mongers behavior is not usually that of a gentleman. In fact, they often treat these women as chattel. Despite this strong call to secrecy and discretion, mongers break their own rules of the game. First, they freely take pictures of sex workers as "personal" memories, most of the time without their consent. Then, they post these pictures in the Internet to be shared by all members.

Moe3333, for example, asks the basic question whether the sex workers allow the pictures to be taken: "Do the ladies of costa rica allow you to take pics usually? Do you have to pay extra or how does all that work? If they let you take some pics, what kind of pics? clothed? in the act? you know what im getting at ?"[17] Koppite answers back that some like it and some don't. Nevertheless, the majority does not want the pictures to be in the Internet: "Just ask–each chica has a different attitude towards pictures –some dont like them at all– some are ok with fully clothed and some will allow '*sin ropas*' Most however will try and insist on no internet posting of any photos."[18] Superman thinks most of them pose for free and some even send their pictures later. "Every girl i've asked have gladly posed, shoot one girl even took my address and sent me more photo's of herself!"[19]

For Bilko, if women object to having their pictures taken, money can make the trick: "Just to add my experiences, about 2/3 have no problem with nude pics. half of the rest want no pics at all. A small number want money, you can decide if they are worth the extra few dollars."[20]

Don Giovanni promises his pictures are only "para mis recuerdos únicamente" and he convinces sex workers to let him take the pictures with his advanced technology: " I showed the girls the results on the LCD monitor. Several of the girls became enthused and began posing like models, and I was able to coax them into removing their clothes in the process. I was with 6 different woman, and have nude photos of 5 of them."[21]

Bombero, on the other hand, sees things differently. According to him, the women are now more apprehensive about the picture taking. He suggests that some mongers are revealing to the women where the pictures end up in Internet and in doing so, are showing them what happens in what may considered 'secret' events like a bachelor's party.

> *indeed, girls are more apprehensive about fotos than ever. I was refused fotos even with their clothes on outside the hotel . . . according to one, she didn't want them on the internet although she didn't say crt specifically. That guy capo saw at the del Buey reminds me of the guy in your group that tells all the girls what transpires at the bachelor party. he does it because he has no game other than that.*[22]

Despite such promises, the reality is that the men would not abide by them.

Let's see how Sasha is "shared" by the registered users of CostaRicaticas.com: Pinellasguy confesses he found her picture in the Internet and thinks "she looks tremendously hot to my eyes. Anybody out there have any experience with her? Should she be on my to do list.?"[23] WillySp respons that Sasha is "A definite on the to do list. Sasha provides a fantastic experience. Great massage and I had the pleasure of giving her a massage as well."[24] Texcdu supports her very strongly and tells other mongers that the woman is "great as 3some with Paola."[25] Koppite recalls he had the woman for his anniversary party and he thinks, "*She is muy caliente.*" Pelo de Gato says that Sasha works better in "threesomes with Erica, Brenda and Jennifer."[26] Scubabum advises his prospective clients to make her provide oral sex as she is "the second best head I ever had."[27] DelBuey Dave is in full agreement: "She gives one of the best BJ's that I have ever had. She's just plain great at it."[28] For Astroglide, "This girl gets the trophy for phuck of the year. Her attitude should be bottled and sold for cien a bottle. I don't know how she pulls it off, but it seems like each guy is her *favorito* . . . and she knows her job is to make you feel like you are the freaking king. I know this is just a job for her . . . but she would NEVER let on, even on a bad day. She is that good."[29]

CapoD2T recognizes that mongers do not keep their promises. But he thinks the big problem is that some of them tell the women where their pictures are being shown. Those who reveal this information are disloyal to their buddies:

> *Why someone would do that I have no idea but it happens. I recently saw a guy bring a chica over to the monitor in the Del Buey, and show her CRT . . . I do not butt in and I did not know the guy, so I have no idea if he was a member, a VIP or what, but he did it was not the VIP section but the site itself and it was something to do with photos as the conversation ensued.... Whoever it was, was he trying to be a big shot in front of the ladies or whatever I think that is in incredibly poor taste and an insult to us all. I am not a confrontational person nor was it any of my business, to say something, so I kept quiet but I was sitting typing an email next to him when he did it.. pretty phucked up if you ask me . . . . !*[30]

Snooky is so upset by such disloyalty that he suggests punishments against the "moles.": "You should have noted his screen name (next to the logout button) and shot an e–mail to the admin telling him that "so and so" was phucking up our world."[31]

Mighty1 has moral doubts about whether or not the promises should be kept. He believes that one should respect one's agreements and that if a monger promises not to show the pictures, he should not do it later. Nevertheless, he rationalizes some monger's behaviors by indicating that the pictures are shown only in the VIP section of their websites, a place for future customers: "The *chicas* are concerned about their privacy and well they should be but the pictures are on a secured location for people who have paid a membership so VIP members should realize that by letting all this out all they are doing is ruining it for all of us. If you promise a *chica* that you won't post a picture –I feel you should honor that but otherwise it is fair game. I did happen to get pictures but it was with some persuading on my part– It also helped that I gave them some nice t–shirts to wear and pose. Somehow that really got them comfortable!"[32]

Anyone who registers as a member and pays a small fee to a sex news group, can have access to the VIP section. Shasha, for example, is shown in some pictures providing oral sex; in other pictures, she is having anal sex and vaginal sex with one, two and three different men. If these pictures are printed, Sasha can be taken to court and lose custody over her children and be fired from her day job as a receptionist. This suggests that her privacy and health are not the main monger's concern. It is one of the major failures of monger culture that fail to protect these women who provide so much love and pleasure.

Notes

1. http://www.costaricaticas.com/phpbb2/viewtopic.php?t=1725
2. http://www.costaricaticas.com/phpbb2/viewtopic.php?t=3468
3. http://www.costaricaticas.com/phpbb2/viewtopic.php?t=988
4. http://www.costaricaticas.com/phpbb2/viewtopic.php?t=988
5. http://www.costaricaticas.com/phpbb2/viewtopic.php?t=988
6. http://www.costaricaticas.com/phpbb2/viewtopic.php?t=988
7. http://www.costaricaticas.com/phpbb2/viewtopic.php?t=988
8. http://www.costaricaticas.com/phpbb2/viewtopic.php?t=988
9. http://www.costaricaticas.com/phpbb2/viewtopic.php?t=988
10. http://www.costaricaticas.com/phpbb2/GeneralInformation
11. http://www.costaricaticas.com/phpbb/GeneralInformation
12. J. Davidson O'Connell, "British Sex Tourists in Thailand," in M. Maynard and J. Purvis (eds) (Hetero) *Sexual Politics,* Lodon: Taylor and Francis, 1995.
13. J. Seabrook, *Travels in the Skin Trade: Tourism and the Sex Industry,* London: Pluto Press, 1996, pp. 114–115.
14. http://www.costaricaticas.com/phpbb2/GeneralInformation
15. http://www.costaricaticas.com/phpbb/GeneralInformation
16. http://www.costaricaticas.com/phpbb2/viewtopic.php?t=2927
17. http://www.costaricaticas.com/phpbb2/viewtopic.php?t=3543
18.
19. http://www.costaricaticas.com/phpbb2/viewtopic.php?t=3543
20. http://www.costaricaticas.com/phpbb2/viewtopic.php?t=3543
21. http://www.costaricaticas.com/phpbb2/viewtopic.php?t=3543
22. http://www.costaricaticas.com/phpbb2/viewtopic.php?t=3543
23. http://www.costaricaticas.com/phpbb2/viewtopic.php?t=3664

24. http://www.costaricaticas.com/phpbb2/viewtopic.php?t=3664
25. http://www.costaricaticas.com/phpbb2/viewtopic.php?t=3664
26. http://www.costaricaticas.com/phpbb2/viewtopic.php?t=3664
27. http://www.costaricaticas.com/phpbb2/viewtopic.php?t=3543
28. http://www.costaricaticas.com/phpbb2/viewtopic.php?t=3664
29. http://www.costaricaticas.com/phpbb2/viewtopic.php?t=3664
30. http://www.costaricaticas.com/phpbb2/viewtopic.php?t=3543
31. http://www.costaricaticas.com/phpbb2/viewtopic.php?t=3543
32. http://www.costaricaticas.com/phpbb2/viewtopic.php?t=3543

12. Lying and Simulation

One of the tenets of sexual education in Costa Rica is the importance of honesty and the ability to tell the truth. [1] It is assumed that when you state what you want and are able to listen to the other's needs, there is a better chance to negotiate, compromise and avoid doing harm to each other. This ideal is far removed from the reality of the Gulch. In the sex tourism industry, whatever idea we might have of the truth, is not part of the culture. People are expected there to lie through their teeth.

PacoLoco, for example, can never detect when the women are telling the truth. He asked: "I met a hot *chica* at the Blue Queen, she claimed it was her first night there and I felt like I was taking advantage of her for 30k so I gave her *cien*. She calls me "*mi amor*", kisses me and makes me feel special, so I really think she is in love with me. But our "dates" always end up with her asking for more money at the end of the night. I saw her again at the BM after she said she didn't work there anymore and she told me she was just hanging with her friends. Could this girl be lying to me? Should I give her the $1000.00 she says she needs for school?" [2]

Captain cannot believe Pacoloco might be so naive. He cracks up with the question and says that "I'm lying here, 3 days after being sliced and diced to repair a double hernia, and both Paco and Latino are doing their best to bust my stitches wide open." [3] Astroglide, finally, reveals to Pacoloco the stark truth: sex workers are lying to him and if he does not believe it, he should consult "the experts":

> *You will meet many hot chicas in Costa Rica. With very few exceptions, they will all be lying to you. In the Blue Queen Bar, the will ALL be lying to you. On that rare occasion when you find the newbie there for her first night, do a little due diligence before being taken in by her story. Check her scorecard with Vegas*

Bob who should be lurking nearby. Chances are he has already done her, and knows all the other guys that did her as well. Never pay cien . . . and never pay what they ask for . . . andif you pay MORE than what they ask for you may be killed by other CRT members. [4]

Astroglide also warned PacoLoco that another big lie sex workers proclamations of love. He advised PacoLoco not to believe what they may say to him :

They always call you "mi amor." That means "stupid gringo asshole" in espaniol. They are very good at making you thinking they really love you. If they did, they would never bring up money. By asking for more money at the end of the night she is proving what she REALLY sees in you . . . a big fat walking ATM card. Don't be that stupid. [5]

Finally, sex workers will lie about their work. Some say that they are no longer in the business and if they happen to be at Del Buey, it is to visit their female friends. Astroglide does not buy it:

No chica hangs out at the BM with her friends unless she is "on the program" the Hotel Del Buey is well known by EVERY chica in Costa Rica . . . as well as most chicas in every central american city. Once a chica starts "working" at the hotel Del Buey, they are lost . . . ruined . . . destroyed. Oh, we can still screw them, but they are worthless as far as any emotional honesty is concerned. So to answer your question, I guarantee she is lying to you. [6]

Lying is so endemic that Pacoloco does not even believe the woman's age. PacoLoco wants to know whether there is another time conception, such as the one proposed by the phenomenologists: "I recently met a sweet, affectionate Colombiana at Tea Amargo, she made eyes at me, blew kisses from across the room, and called me *"mi amor*" within 1 minute of our introductions. I knew for sure this was "the one", it was truly love at first sight, or so I thought. We drank, danced then made love for many minutes in my hotel room (for an agreed price). She claimed she was 26, but my amigo asked if that was in "DelBuey Years?" Can you explain DelBuey years? Is that somehow related to "Tica–time"?" [7]

According to Astroglide, the question has been asked many times before. He does indeed recognize that sex workers have changed the traditional conception of clock–time. Your Del Buey age is not the same as your chronological age:

Many have asked me that question, and I am happy to explain it here. A "Del Buey Year" refers to the amount of time a chica claims to age, while working at the Del Buey. A "Del Buey Year" is actually three years for every year claimed.

In other words, if your 26 year old Columbiana started working at the Del Buey when she was 20, and she told you she was 26, she would really be 38, because she was claiming only one year for every three years working there. It is very difficult to know for sure, because most latina's look younger than they really are. For example, Lucy, a well known Del Buey puta, is actually 110. She doesn't look a day over 60. In her earlier years she was known to have had a steamy affair with Pancho Villa. [8]

Astroglide continues: "On the same token, if a *Tica* tells you to wait for her, she will be back in one hour, it will probably be more like two hours, or not at all. *Tica* time is never definite, always an estimate, and always a lie. *Ticas* feel no obligation to follow any certain time. Most of them love to be given a watch but rarely wear one, and never look at one. If the estimate given is for the FOLLOWING day, the chances are in the 90% range that by the following morning, the promise to show up will have been completely forgotten. *Ticas* have no guilt or shame about this. In fact, it is expected. If a *Tica* does show up on time, it is obviously a mistake." [9]

Americans, on the other hand, have a strong loyalty to clock time. If PacoLoco makes an appointment with Astroglide to meet at 2 pm., is to be expected both men will be on time.) This is the reason they usually get mad at sex workers, since they are usually late. They think this is a sign of lack of maturity and honesty.

But are mongers really that honest with regard to time?

Monger themselves have a different conception of time and their age is also generally altered. In fact, most of them are honest about their age only until they reach the 60's. Moerkerk, for example, is seventy–one but claims to be sixty–three; Palotieso is 80 years old but told Jackeline he was 70 years old. "I saw his passport and found out his true age," she said. "Don Paco says he is in his late fifties" –Juanita stated– "but I think he means the 1850's." Rachel discovered that Hardcore was not in the Viet Nam War, as he claimed, but in World War II. "He thinks I am stupid –she added– because he showed me a picture in black and white and told me that it was taken in Viet Nam. He thinks I don't know there were color films already in the 1970's."

Not only do they claim to be younger, but they also stretch the time when it is in their interest to do so: "Yes, it is related to Tica Time. Tica Time is generally double to triple the equivalent in Monger Time. A monger hour is actually slightly less than an hour, around 43 minutes. If a monger claims he screwed a chica non–stop for 30 minutes, it was probably more like 14."

If VegasBob cannot come in an hour with Sasha, she tells us that the man hides his watch and convinces her that "We still have twenty minutes left." When Natasha agrees with John34 on $500 for a week at the beach, he later tries to make her believe that a week implies from Monday to Monday instead of Monday to Friday.

Do mongers also lie to sex workers?

Sex workers are not the only ones that lie; mongers also do not disclose their names, profession, and place of origin, marriage status, age or income. The advice they give to each other on the sex boards is never to reveal one's background, as this might lead to extortions and blackmail. There are also rumors in the Forums that the FBI is monitoring websites and that the Costa Rican Government is following their information to crack down on pimping. Vegas Bob, Astroglide or Pacoloco not only hide their true identity in the sex forums, but also in their interactions with sex workers. They only use their first name, usually a pseudonym, and their last name is seldom shared. It is very rare that they provide their mail address to a sex worker and when they communicate with her, they do it only through email. Home phone numbers are only given to their "*novias* and this is rather the exception." As of income, they lie about their earning power as this might lead sex workers to demand more money.

Mongers lie about their activities in Costa Rica. First of all, they have as a rule never to tell an American woman what they do in Costa Rica.

> *We have all kinds of rules about our behavior in Costa Rica that are discussed on this board. But we do not have any for our behavior back home. So I will submit some new rules for behavior in the real world.*
>
> *No. 1: Never tell a female what you do in Costa Rica.*
>
> *No. 2: Never tell a male who may tell a female.*
>
> *No. 3: If rule No. 1 or No. 2 or broken deny it and stick to that story.*[10]

Goal does not only hide it from female friends but also from his male friends who come together to Costa Rica: "Hell I even took a office buddy with me last trip and didn't tell him shit. He did the rainforest tour and we went to dinner but I didn't show him Delray or any MP's."[11]

Jazz Musician wants to have a committed relationship with a sex worker, but also wants to be unfaithful. He asks other sex tourists whether he should tell her the truth or not.

> *You've got a girl who's very into you and it's mutual. You go down to see her but you only have a couple days. You want to do the TLN thing with her (as does she), but you'd like to get out for a few hours during the days.*
> *You:*
> *1.) Tell her the truth*

2.) Make up some complicated story involving an amigo(s)
3.) Give it up. You're married.
4.) Suggest a three–some
5.) Phuck it; disappear for a few hours– went jogging
6.) Other [12]

PacoLoco believes that telling the truth should never be an option. He suggests it is better to ask for a threesome. [13] The rest suggest he should lie. Depanz1 proposes to him to send the woman to get her nails done. He also includes a mantra that indicates how he stands with regard to asking questions: "ASK ME NO QUESTIONS, I TELL YOU NO LIES." [14] Tman proposes a good excuse: "Develop some "business interests"...thats always the Latin acceptable excuse to be absent . . . . [15] Papa Nut also thinks the truth should not be told. It is better to give free money than to state honesty the sexual desires:

> *Wow, a mongers dilemma. What ever you do, don't let her know your going for a little strange. Chica's are a very jealous breed. She'll have an idea of what's going on. After all, you are in SJO. Best suggestion was to give her a little spending money for the mall. Tell her to buy a special outfit for the evening festivities, then put her in a cab. Guaranteed to buy you several hour's of play-time.* [16]

Latinoheat69 also goes for the lie: "Send her ass home for the afternoon to tend to her K*ds." [17]

Astroglide tries to explain the women's behavior. First, he does not blame them because to "understand the *chica* mentality you have to look at the way they were raised." According to him, "From an early age they are thought to USE their sexuality to get what they want. Most of them have no fathers in the home. They learn about males from their Tico boyfriends."

"These fine gentlemen –he continues– train our latinas that they are good for one thing . . . screwing. They teach them if they want something, they gotta flaunt their sexuality." This is the reason, for him, that the women are such liers: "They learn to lie, cheat, and steal to survive. They learn that the sluttier they dress, the more attention they get." Macho Latino men –adds Astroglide– have taught sex workers "the prettier they are, the better chance they have of getting what they want. They learn that turning it on and off is just a game. They learn that the *Ticos* they are taught by really will never love them for them, but only for those short encounters of sexual activity. These encounters are usually uninspired, and over quickly . . . and the Tico moves on to his next *chica*."

So, the guilty party is Latin men who make women "take this attitude to the Del Buey, and use all they have learned against helpless gringos that do not know how to play the game. These gringos become putty in their hands and are easily abused. Sadly, some of them like it that way, but the smart ones wise up, and learn to play the game. Hopefully, so will you." [18] American men, who are the ones who buy sex from them, are not the ones responsible for prostitution. They treat women –according to him– as human beings and do not teach them that the "the pu*sy is their most powerful device, and it can be used to get almost anything."

But is this difference between American and Latin men really true? Do mongers treat these women differently from Latino men or is this just another big lie?

Most sex workers think that American men do not play fair. María, for example, thinks that they appear more romantic and sensitive but "This stops at the airport. They make the whole affair a big lie. Once in America, whatever was promised is forgotten." She recalls a romance with a monger who told her he was totally in love with her. He also indicated that he was divorced and that he would send for her to the States. "I am still waiting. PacoLoco told me that the man has been married for forty years!!!" –she adds. Liliana was given a credit card and a ticket to go to Miami. "The credit card bounced three hours after he left the country. The ticket was forged," she confesses. María got the first installment of the money Palotieso promised her for her education. "I got a letter the second month that stated Palotieso had had a heart attack and was unable to send more money. Three months later she sees him at Del Buey with two of her girlfriends."

The women also resent the American men's intolerance toward their social manners. Anita tells us that she is tired of being told not to speak loudly and to laugh less. "PepeGordo is always hushing me and telling me to quiet down. He thinks I am too vulgar." Miriam resents being told to close her mouth when eating and to use the knive and fork in the same manner as the monger does. Gretel hates when her clients tell her not to drink so much beer and want her to drink wine instead. Talía believes it is an invasion of her privacy when the client gives her advice on the amount of perfume she should wear. Rita does not like when she is told to stop dressing like a whore.

Sex tourists also frequently turn violent. Shasha is forced by some of her clients to have oral sex for very long periods of time. "I hate to do this for more than 10 minutes and when I tell the client to rush, he gets very upset. There have been times when I am forced to continue." Penélope shows us scars she has from customers who were violent to her. "Don Pepe hit me when I told him that I would not see him anymore." Rita confesses she's had more than one black eye from customers who wanted to have sex more than once for the same price.

American sex tourists differ from Latin men only in the intensity searched during short periods of time. Lucrecia thinks that her local relationships are less into communicating and more into doing things together. "American tourists talk too much. They want to analyze everything and they want to share their life stories. Latin men, on the other hand, prefer to do things together, such as dancing or listening to music. They don't want to share their feelings as much as the gringos."- She concludes. Rita also thinks that the differences are not that great. "Gringos can be very rude sometimes. They think that we Latinos are inferior, whether they admit it or not. They talk to us like children and they think they come here to lecture us in how to live our lives. This is the same shit men do, be Latinos or gringos"- she adds.

Mongers and sex workers also lie about their sexual practices. Sex workers conceal the number of clients they have, the number of times they have done unsafe sex and the diversity of sexual practices they have engaged in. Anita never admits, "I have had a client prior to the current one, as this disappoints the client." She tells her clients that she always uses condoms, something she seldom does. "I can charge more when the customer thinks I am making him the exception." Sex tourists also lie about the number of sex workers they have had sex with. They perceive Latin prostitutes as jealous and inquisitive about their activities. They report that the women even check whether they ejaculate or not. "If they see no juice, they get mad –says Jack52– and demand an explanation." For these reasons, sex tourists do not acknowledge the number of "*novias*" or "friends" with whom they engage in bareback sex.

The Gulch is a culture based on many lies. It is not the type of community where the traditional educational interventions, based on sexual communication and honesty, might have a positive impact. Several sex workers who are infected hide the fact from their clients. It is also expected the men would do the same.

Sex tourists usually call Costa Rica a new Disneyworld. It is an eroticized place for seniors to play games not easily attainable in the United States. This is not new since from the 19th Century Europeans have erotized women of different cultures and races, whereby their sexuality was defined as highly attractive and fascinating, yet relegated to the natural primitiveness and lower order of the other cultural group. According to Roy Porter, exotic lands and peoples provided Europeans with "paradigms of the erotic." Away from the repressive sexual mores of Western Europe, different cultures and particularly the women in them became sites where sex "was neither penalized, not pathologized nor exclusively procreative." [19]

It looks like fun from a distance but once you look closer, the place is more like a war zone.

Both Jeff and María pretend to be something they are not. Since she is not an innocent child who looks for someone to teach her what her place should be and Jeff is not the charming prince who is to rescue her from poverty and underdevelopment, their relationship is distorted and untrue from the beginning.

Costa Rica is no Disneyworld. Jeff would see María a few times after their first encounter at Del Buey and send her –after his return trip– a nice postcard from the States. In his next trip, he will not call her anymore. There are too many hot women at the hotel to waste time on one. María, on the other hand, would start having sex as soon as Jeff is on the plane. If Costa Rica is Disneyworld; Snow White is having sex with all the dwarves.

Astroglide warns other mongers not to be fooled by how the place seems to them.

> *I am not the first guy to compare CR to Disneyworld. I just caution that everything you see there is NOT always as it seems. When you start believing that it is real . . . . I worry that you can then slip into an emotional weakness that can be damaging later. Guard your heart. Most of the time the chicas you meet at the Del Buey are really good manipulators and you can get burned.* [20]

The American sex tourist is aware that the sex scene is a simulation. Simulation is different from lying; it is more a theatrical act than a denial of a known fact. When you simulate feelings and desires, you might not be actually lying, as there is room for self–delusion. Simulation sometimes becomes so "real" than it is no longer possible to know whether it is true or not. As opposed to lying, no single fact unveils a well–performed act of simulation.

Because simulation is never black or white, both sex workers and mongers become obsessed with finding whatever truth remains in the performance.

Sex workers are never sure whether these men really mean what they say. Do mongers want a long–term relationship when they act as "*caballeros*" and loving and nurturing men? If they do not want commitments, why talk about them?

Lucy says that many men have promised her marriage and a life in the United States. Some might mean it at the time, but once they return home, "Mongers forget everything they promised." Margarita was never sent the ticket that Charles promised. Lupe says she is still hoping that Peter will marry her but "he keeps postponing." Gretel was left waiting at the airport as her American lover changed his mind at the last minute and took an earlier flight. Miriam agreed to have her pictures taken as the man wanted to show them to his family. She eventually found them in Internet with an inscription that said: "Miriam gives the best blow–jobs in town."

If all mongers were like those mentioned above, then sex workers would have total certainty of their ill intentions. Nevertheless, like in any gamble, some women get "lucky" and find love and marriage. There are only a few but this is enough to give hope to others. "Carmen was able to marry and move to Florida –says Conchita– and I hope I will be able too." When we told her that

Carmen was the exception to the rule, Conchita did not want to hear it: "I like to play the lottery and I know one day I will hit the jackpot."

American male tourists are also obsessed in figuring out sex workers' intentions. Despite a hunch that the women are acting, there is some self–delusion that they might not be.

In one of the forums, the discussion revolved around whether or not women sex workers are faking their orgasms. Some, like Papa Nut, believed sex workers faked them in order to please their clients: "Because they think we care." [21] Goetzvonberlishingen thinks he is an expert in spotting women who fake their orgasms and gives recommendations on how to discover them. Nevertheless, he later concedes that it is rather irrelevant whether they are true or not.

> *How do you know they are faking? Of course a poor performance is obvious, but when I have them bucking and screaming and generally going wild and I check the source of all glory and it is soaking wet with their boiled okra slime like leche which by the way has a very distinct taste, I can be pretty sure that the chica came for real. Also the sweat and heartbeat have a different feel and smell than just "exercise" would produce. If the ones I know are faking it then they have developed a superhuman control of the autonomic nervous system. But if you believe it, who cares? It's like the whole experience, if you get what you want and your fantasy is intact, does it really matter if it is real or fake, as long as it is real to you? I just want more time and subjects for research. Maybe we could run ph tests and specific gravity tests, etc on the juices and develop a template for determining fake versus real orgasms, maybe even develop a field test strip like the narcs have for opiates, but come to think of it the only place that would have a market would be in gringa land and then, once again, who cares? Pura vida,* [22]

Joe1015 laughs at this expert on orgasms: "that is ph*cking hilarious! can you picture us halfway into a session, then stopping abruptly to taste her vaginal secretions and then inserting a 'ph strip' into her vagina to confirm a true orgasm?" [23] Goetz does not fool himself: "The answer is simple, they fake it in hopes of getting you to come faster." [24] Sooky thinks is a matter of money: "But since it is free for them, these are probably mockeries: "If they were paying for it and not visa versa MAYBE we'd care. NAHHH" [25]

Despite this behavior, sex workers can also enjoy sex with some customers and can also grow fond of them. Therefore, it is also hard for mongers to know for sure who is simulating an orgasm and who is not. They expect the worst but hope for the best.

After much deliberation, American males admit that they will never know what is real in the sex worker's hearts and minds. Sex workers also would not be able to tell which customers can end up being their saviors and which ones will just use them for a while.

In another thread, the discussion is about the reality of the tears shed at airports by prostitutes when the American "*novio*" leaves. "Are the tears real?" –Pocoloco asks. "Why fake them?"

> *Now here is the question . . . Do the tears stop the minute you get out of the taxi or turismo and do they head right back to their place of work and get right back on the white horse . . . or are the tears for real and they are truly herfelt and not able to function for several days before they head back to work . . . 26*

Texcdn argues that the tears could be real but it is impossible to tell.

> *I think people (men and women) can turn on the waterworks for different reasons:*
>
> *1. "At that moment" they actually feel sad. They could be sad, because they genuinely had a good time with you. I think that many of the women fall into this camp. Sure they are motivated by the money, but look at it from a personal perspective. I work at my job for the money, period. I prefer employment opportunities where I also enjoy what I do. I think the same could be said for them. If they have a good time with a guy, it makes the day–to–day work more palatable.*
>
> *2. "Academy award" –These people are more cunning. They sense that a guy wants them to cry, and they will do whatever they need to in order to hit the heartstrings. These are the more dangerous ones!* [27]

Californication believes they are real but for different reasons: "They are genuinely crying as they think to themselves, 'Damn it now i have to go buy a new long distance phone card'. These broads are cheap and don't like to spend a dime." [28] ElObispo, with humor, agrees with him: "The only reason they go to the airport with you is to check out the men on the incoming flights." [29]

Mighty1 advises mongers to enjoy the tears while they last.

> *Who really cares what they do once they leave? The important thing to realize here is that at least they are there to see you off. If they cry and get emotional, so much the more it feeds the GFFE (Girlfriend Fantasy Experience). Once they are gone –they may still feel emotional or not but to me– out of sight, out of mind. It is the next guy's turn to get her.*
> *Guys, enjoy the ride and realize that it ends at some point and yes somebody else gets their turn on this ride but find comfort in the fact that at least you had a turn.* [30]

The answers to these questions are not simple. Sex workers admit that they fake their orgasms most of the time and that sex work is simply work for them. They have a capacity to shut down the experience and detach very easily from it: "I am thinking of the errands I have to do in the morning" –says Karina about what goes on in her mind when she is having sex with a customer. "I don't feel anything"– she adds.

Don Giovanni is aware that sex tourism is what Baudrilliard calls "simulacra", an event that seems so real that the person no longer cares whether it is true or not:

> *Some GFs have cried when I left, and kept in touch afterwards. I know many of you insist this is all an illusion based on greed, lies and deception. Almost assuredly, you are correct, but I really don't care. I think of the old 1970s song that goes something like: "If it feels this good being used, you can use me up." I still keep a positive checking and savings account, and put the maximum in my 401K, so the money I spend on Ticas is really insignificant in the overall scheme of things, and has been well worth it.* [31]

The problem with "simulacra" is that to keep the fantasies alive, people will distort whatever contradicts them. According to Baudrilliard in postmodern America, there is no longer any "reality" left to make a comparison between the real and the faked. It is no longer relevant to say the real world "exists" and hence no system of representation or analysis can refer to it as such. This philosopher would argue that mongers should not worry whether sex workers simulate or not, as simulation is as real as it can get. [32]

Nevertheless, mongers know that there is a "real" life in Costa Rica that is unknown to them. Yet despite this awareness, it is not sought after since the men want no part in it.

American sex tourists show a tendency of not wanting to see any "truth" when they deny the reality of breast implants. According to a self–taken poll, most of them do not like silicone and prefer "home grown." [33] DBCocker says that the women who had surgery would be very disappointed to see this survey, as American tourists do not like it: "Imagine what all the chicas with blown up tits would say if they saw this survey." [34] Buzz comments that the results would anger more the Colombianas, as most of them have opted for the operation: "You would destroy some of the columbianas (sic) the way this is going!" [35]

Nevertheless, most women who are professional sex workers have had the operation. This surgery delivers more money to sex workers as the interviewee themselves confirm that they earn more since their breast augmentation's operation. So, either the sex tourists cannot tell when a woman has silicone breasts (very unlikely as they themselves admit not liking the feeling of them) or they shun the reality and pretend, once again, not to know.

Another sign that there is a tendency to escape from a crude reality is the monger's inversion of women's personalities. These men seem to feel a need to see the world upside down: mongers describe American women as selfish and materialistic prostitutes whereas Latin sex workers are portrayed as sensitive, caring and loving human beings. It is somehow perplexing that the woman who does not charge is the one who is portrayed as a prostitute.

Tman, for example, believes that it is the American woman the one who is truly a sex worker. According to him, "the American or jewish princesses normally have only one mode . . . consumerism and financial security." Their material greed, he continues, is responsible for their lack of eroticism: "Sex and other matters come way down the list for these types." It is American culture that is responsible since it "causes so many layers of guilt, repression and anxiety that it is surprising ANY of us can get it up anymore." Given the fact that sex is "dead" in the States, "Thank God for the discovery of the basic latin culture and the ladies that come from it . . . which helps us recover some of our innocence lost. My eyes are getting misty as I write this . . . ."[36]

The perception that paid sex is really free and that free sex is really paid, leads to other denials. The first one is semantic, as mongers do not feel comfortable in calling sex workers "whores." The term is too "derogatory." Furthermore, most mongers hope that behind the desire for money, sex workers genuinely care for them.

> *In sum, I think what the labels denote are technically accurate, but what they connote is another story. .. In general, I would never refer to a chica as a whore, particularly to her face, because of the negative connotations, unless I felt particular actions qualified her for that label. For example, if she made our session all about the money by insisting on the money upfront, upselling her services and cutting out early after barely performing what she was paid for or if she acted like providing that service was the worst thing she would want to do. Needless to say, I do not run into many girls like that in CR, but they are out there. More so at the DB, land of the $100 fixed rate. The funny thing is very often it is the chica that goes for the lower rate that provides the better service and does not act at all like a whore. My last comment is that, as far as using the term whore, I would be as likely or more to use it to refer to a non–prostitute gringa who plays men who she is not really interested in except for the material things he provides –money, jewelry, dinner, clothes etc.*[37]

Costa Rican sex workers should never be called "whores" when they are "honest about their feelings toward you, never play games with your emotions, never asked you for money and are happy with what you gave them and still let you be a man." Tman knows some will not agree with him. Nevertheless, "For those of you who say that 'whores will always be whores', well . . . it may well be true but there is always that exception to the rules. I know many guys who are still happily married to former prostitutes and many that are not. Just my 2 cents worth."[38]

Prolijo admits that these women are technically "whores," but he still thinks the term is not fair to them and that he would not use it.

> *In sum, I think what the labels denote are technically accurate, but what they connote is another story. .. In general, I would never refer to a chica as a whore, particularly to her face, because of the negative connotations, unless I felt particular actions qualified her for that label. For example, if she made our session all about the money by insisting on the money upfront, upselling her services and cutting out early after barely performing what she was paid for or if she acted like providing that service was the worst thing she would want to do.*[39]

Kamala Kempadoo in her study on Caribbean sex tourism finds the same pattern of denial. She believes that there is a cultural misunderstanding that misreads signs:

> *Yet for tourists from cultures where in hegemonic discourse sexuality symbolizes love and desire, and is considered to be sullied by economic relations, especially for women, flirtations and solicitations from young women and men are easily read as signs of nonprostitution activities that approximate genuine interest and attraction.*[40]

Similar to the Costa Rican mongers, Kempadoo finds that sex tourists in the Caribbean do not to see sex workers exclusively as that but as genuine companions. On a "World Sex Guide" website eighty–three letters were written by sex tourists about the Caribbean who indicated that most or all of the sex workers were "not real hookers." While accepting that women participated in prostitution due to financial need and a lack of other economic opportunities, the letters stressed that the men believed that the women genuinely enjoyed all types of sex with them, and that the women were particularly good at what they did.[41]

This leads mongers to deny that money plays an overwhelming role in the sex workers' actions. Sex tourists do not feel comfortable speaking or dealing with the money directly with the sex worker. Mongers will usually pay indirectly like placing the money in the sex workers purse or leaving the money in a drawer or an envelope. This becomes confusing as the women are made to look for it and to guess where it is, something that promotes stealing. Prolijo is aware the reason behind this behavior is to hide there is a commercial exchange:

> *Most of us feel slightly uncomfortable discussing the money issues for one reason or another. Perhaps it is because it brings home the fact that the whole thing is really just a commercial exchange rather than the GFFE we would prefer to pretend. I don't know. But it is really much better to suck it up and make things clear before you leave the bar, particularly if hotel chica fees are involved, but if for no other reason than to avoid any unnecessary unpleasantness.* [42]

Another subject the American tourists do not want to deal with is the sex worker's living situation. Most of them are shocked when they venture into the women's neighborhoods and homes. They admit that in the United States they would never enter such slums.

Astroglide recognizes that most mongers do not visit the sex worker's family. Apparently, this will show them the poor conditions shared by its members. He tells mongers to do it at least once in their lifetime, not because they could do something to improve the woman's lot, but to "simulate a real interest in her." Astroglide recognizes that most mongers do not visit the sex worker's family. Nevertheless, he recommends that "If you can . . . go home with them." [43]

"Why bother?"- He asks.

He explains that in his last trip his girlfriend asked him to come to meet his mother. For him " this was a real eye opening experience" since it allowed him to see "The little shack where she lives. She has no bed, but sleeps on the floor." Her mother turned to be friendly and when he asked whether he could sleep with her daughter she said "*No hay problema*": He continues. "I expressed surprise at that and she said every other guy she has ever brought home her mother disliked. Me, she liked. Now I know that was because I was a rich gringo in her eyes, but still, the opportunity is there. I really may do it on my next trip over there. The problem is . . . my babe can get loud something, so I hope she doesn't wake momma! Also, I have not slept on the floor since I was in boy scouts." [44] When one visits sex workers' homes, concludes Astroglide, "the sex gets much, much better. One should simulate an interest in the woman's life to spice up the fucking." [45]

Mongers want to believe that prostitutes are honest women who care for them. Any financial demand, no matter how small, is perceived as a refutation of this belief. Astroglide, for example, is pretty sensitive about being "scammed," though he knows this will eventually happen. His coping strategy if he is asked for money is to leave the woman and move to the next one. Multiple rejections help him avoid deception: "But the wonderful thing about this "search" for the *gfe* is that as soon as you get tired, bored, or sense that she is scamming you . . . you just pick up and move on." [46]

Finally, Mexpat admits that too much contact is not his favorite hobby as he finds out something he wants not to see: he has nothing in common with the women he dates.

> *Sure, I could have gotten involved in a "relationship" with some chica if I had really wanted to. There are plenty around looking for a meal ticket. But the problem with speaking pretty good Spanish and understanding Latin cultures to some extent is that you quickly realize that 90% of these available chicas are really, really dull. They are largely uneducated, ignorant and for the most part, emotionally irrational and childish.* [47]

Sex tourism leads people to "fantasy–land" where sex workers are caring and unselfish, easy to please, and real potential partners back home are materialistic and selfish. Men who otherwise are smart, educated, business –savvy and quite insightful about life in America, become more like children in fairy land, surrounded by beautiful women who help them forget their real obligations back home. This exceptional time lived in the tropics is wonderful for relaxation and fun but it takes them to a mental state of denial that probably goes beyond not wanting to see the sex worker's real lives.

The problem of "fantasy land" is that you see no evil, including HIV.

Notes

1. Johnny Madrigal and Jacobo Schifter, *Encuesta Nacional de Sida*, San José: Asociación Demográfica Costarricense, 1990.
2. http://www.costaricaticas.com/phpBB2/viewtopic.php?t=4615
3. http://www.costaricaticas.com/phpBB2/viewtopic.php?t=4615
4. http://www.costaricaticas.com/phpBB2/viewtopic.php?t=4615
5. http://www.costaricaticas.com/phpBB2/viewtopic.php?t=4615
6. http://www.costaricaticas.com/phpBB2/viewtopic.php?t=4615
7. http://www.costaricaticas.com/phpBB2/viewtopic.php?t=4615
8. http://www.costaricaticas.com/phpBB2/viewtopic.php?t=4615
9. http://www.costaricaticas.com/phpBB2/viewtopic.php?t=4615
10. http://www.costaricaticas.com/phpBB2/viewtopic.php?t=4230
11. http://www.costaricaticas.com/phpBB2/viewtopic.php?t=4230
12. http://www.costaricaticas.com/phpBB2/viewtopic.php?t=4377
13. http://www.costaricaticas.com/phpBB2/viewtopic.php?t=4377
14. http://www.costaricaticas.com/phpBB2/viewtopic.php?t=4377
15. http://www.costaricaticas.com/phpBB2/viewtopic.php?t=4377
16. http://www.costaricaticas.com/phpBB2/viewtopic.php?t=4377
17. http://www.costaricaticas.com/phpBB2/viewtopic.php?t=4377
18. http://www.costaricaticas.com/phpBB2/viewtopic.php?t=4377

19. Roy Porter, "The Exotic as Erotic: Captain Cook in Tahiti," in Roussseaand Porter, *Exotism in the Enlightenment,* edited by G. S.Rousseau and Roy Porter, Manchester University Press, 1990, p. 118.

20. http://216.157.152.197/phpbb2/viewtopic.php?t=4031

21. http://www.costaricaticas.com/phpbb2/viewtopic.php?t=2539

22. http://www.costaricaticas.com/phpbb2/viewtopic.php?t=2539

23. http://www.costaricaticas.com/phpbb2/viewtopic.php?t=2539, http://www.costaricaticas.com/phpbb2/viewtopic.php?t=2539

24. http://www.costaricaticas.com/phpbb2/viewtopic.php?t=3072

25. http://www.costaricaticas.com/phpbb2/viewtopic.php?t=3072

26. http://www.costaricaticas.com/phpbb2/viewtopic.php?t=3072

27. http://www.costaricaticas.com/phpbb2/viewtopic.php?t=3072

28. http://www.costaricaticas.com/phpbb2/viewtopic.php?t=3072

29. http://www.costaricaticas.com/phpbb2/viewtopic.php?t=3072

30. http://www.costaricaticas.com/phpbb2/viewtopic.php?t=3072

31. http://www.costaricaticas.com/phpbb2/viewtopic.php?t=3969

32. Jean Baudrilliard, *Simulacra and Simulation,* Michigan: University of Michigan Press, 1994.

33. http://www.costaricaticas.com/phpBB2/viewtopic.php?t=471

34. http://www.costaricaticas.com/phpBB2/viewtopic.php?t=4717

35. http://www.costaricaticas.com/phpBB2/viewtopic.php?t=4717

36. http://www.costaricaticas.com/phpbb2/viewtopic.php?t=420

37. http://www.costaricaticas.com/phpbb2/viewtopic.php?t=82&postdays=0&postorder=asc&highlight=sending+money&start=15

38. http://www.costaricaticas.com/phpbb2/viewtopic.php?t=82&postdays=0&postorder=asc&highlight=sending+money&start=15

39. http://www.costaricaticas.com/phpbb2/viewtopic.php?t=82&postdays=0&postorder=asc&highlight=sending+money&start=15

40. Kamala Kempadoo, Sexing the Caribbean. Gender, Race and Sexual Labor, London: Routledge, 2004, ebook, p. 2039.

41. Kamala Kempadoo, Sexing the Caribbean. Gender, Race and Sexual Labor, London: Routledge, 2004, ebook, p. 2039.

42. http://www.costaricaticas.com/phpbb2/viewtopic.php?t=82&postdays=0&postorder=asc&highlight=sending+money&start=15

43. http://www.costaricaticas.com/phpbb2/viewtopic.php?t=82&postdays=0&postorder=asc&highlight=sending+money&start=15

44. http://www.costaricaticas.com/phpbb2/viewtopic.php?t=82&postdays=0&postorder=asc&highlight=sending+money&start=15

45. http://www.costaricaticas.com/phpbb2/viewtopic.php?t=82&postdays=0&postorder=asc&highlight=sending+money&start=15

46. http://www.costaricaticas.com/phpbb2/viewtopic.php?t=82&postdays=0&postorder=asc&highlight=sending+money&start=15

47. http://216.157.152.197/phpbb2/viewtopic.php?t=3545

13. The female perspective

Jeff and María had such great sex that they would date several times. After the first night, they would meet again to go out for dinner, to dance and to have more sex. Jeff will show real interest in her story of past sexual abuse and mistreatment by her father and husband number one. She in turn would pay attention to his sad story of divorce and alimony payments that eat away his good salary in the States. During this second date, they would have again passionate sex and have more great conversations in Spanglish. Neither one is very sure that the other understands the story, but the attention seems real in both directions. Three days later, they are still having sex and it is still paid sex. María explains to him that no matter how much she cares for him now, she still needs "the dough" for her children. To prove her point, she makes two concessions: a reduction of the price from $100 to $85 and to have sex without condom.

Money is not the only reason for not using condoms. Sex workers as María do it to establish sexual intimacy with regular clients, "*novios*", lovers or husbands (Tables 11–15–16). Kampadoo found the same pattern in her study on Caribbean sex tourism:

> *For example, whereas many sex working Caribbean women declare that condoms are regularly used with clients, once a client achieves the status of a steady partner, boyfriend or husband, or "man" in a woman's life, condoms are more likely be dispensed with. Sex work is associated with condom use and the likelihood of sexually transmitted diseases, while familiarity is considered safe or healthy.* [1]

According to data from the 2000 survey, sex workers' practices vary between casual and regular clients: 90% of sex workers say that they have had occasional clients who do not want to use condoms. More than 60% admitted having between 1 to 9 casual clients who do not like to use them. (Tables 12–14)

The pattern becomes stronger with regular clients. Sex workers have an average of 11 regular clients a month. Two thirds have between 20 and 50 clients. Despite the fact that 90% indicated they have used the condom during the last sexual relationship, 75% admitted to having between 1 to 9 regular clients who do not want to use them. This means that with regular clients there is a greater chance for unsafe sex. (Table 11)

Apparently, sex workers have different codes of behavior with clients, depending whether they are regular or not. A regular client is anyone who returns more than once. The transition from a casual to a regular client is usually rather quickly. A client might be casual on Monday night and a regular on Wednesday evening, as his return symbolizes a strong liking.

The majority of American tourists like to establish regular relationships with sex workers, a very dangerous practice for unsafe sex. In a Survey in one of the sex forums most mongers admitted that they kept regular relationships.[2]

From sex workers we get information that these regular relationships are dangerous for themselves and also for their clients. Sixty–seven per cent of the sample of sex workers had had sex between 1 and 19 regular clients during the last 30 days. Twenty three per cent had had sex between 20 and 49 regular clients. Most of the sex workers had problems in using condoms with their regular clients. One–third reported no problems with unsafe sex. Forty per cent, on the contrary, recognized having problems in using condoms with one to four of the regular clients. (Table 18)

The search for friendship is evidenced by the many return trips to Costa Rica. 90% of sexual tourists come more than once and one third comes more than ten times. One has been 59 times in the last few years.[3] The more they come the more regular they are perceived by sex workers who get to know them pretty well.

Astroglide, with a sense of humor, starts a thread where many of the tourists admit that Costa Rica, or mongering has become an addiction.

I admit I am addicted to Costa Rica. I spend most of my free time thinking about it, and most of my extra money planning to go back. I just want to warn the newbies (especially those who have not gone down yet) that this place is intoxicating and addictive. I have never smoked cigarettes, and have never experimented with illegal drugs. But I admit I am hooked on this stuff. So, I thought you might be able to list the warning signs, of how you know you have become addicted to Costa Rica:

1. *Everytime you type the word President, you can't stop yourself from adding an E to the end. (Presidente) See, I did it again.*
2. *You wake up hearing the sounds of an old due playing a bad tune on a tuba*

. . . and you are in your own bed.

3. *You go to the mall and every hot babe in a belly shirt you see you wonder if she would be a top earner at the Del Buey.*
4. *You find yourself accidentally answering questions in spanish . . . like at the drive–up window at MacDonalds, when you place your order and add "por favor" at the end, for no apparent reason.*
5. *You are having sex with your wife and accidentally blurt out "Eeeeee, Que Rico."*
6. *You go to the dry cleaners and insist on paying them when they are finished. Forgetting that such has been the policy at every dry cleaners you have ever known.*
7. *After about two months of not being in Costa Rica, you start to get the shakes, and start scratching yourself uncontrollably, everytime you walk by the trojan display at the Drug Store. You then look at them hanging there longingly, and promise to put them out of their misery very soon.*
   You begin to check travelocity.com several times a day, forgetting that you had just checked an hour before. [4]

CapoD2Tcapo adds some more items:

CapoD2TCapo
Joined: 02 Sep 2003
Posts: 136
Location: North Eastern New Jersey
Posted: Sun Jun 13, 2004 9:45 am   Post subject:

Wow I can see this list is going to grow . . .

11. *When you make www.costaricaticas.com your home page.*
12. *When the women at Immigration at San José Airport greets you like an old friend.*
13. *When all the Personal at the El Duende has you on a first name basis and your key is already coded and they no longer need your credit card.*
14. *When all the cast of characters don't bother you anymore as they know your not giving them Shit.*
15. *YOU STOP DATING GRINGAS PERIOD as it is basically a waste of time, effort & Money.*

And the list will grow from here. [5]

Not only do these men travel many times to Costa Rica, but a majority of them even consider relocating to the country. Moving to Costa Rica is for some an escape from America's harsh reality. Men complain that they are fed up of paying mortgages, alimony, and taxes and of the American rat race. They want something peaceful and loving, a place where money is less important. This is rather contradictory as they use money to get it.

It is never clear what are they supposed to get once they move to fairyland. How this new life is meant to be?

McMonger thinks he has found a new Eden on earth. He feels "warmth" in this country and the "smiles" of the "*chicas*" that makes it enticing. This third world country seems so nice and perfect that the man is ready to make the move.

> *After my recent trip to paradise, like many of you guys had indicated, I too certainly experienced that feeling of loss, heartache, and general all around malaise, common to all returning mongers.*
> *All that I experienced, from the warmth of the people, the beauty of the country, and of course the chicas to die for, have caused acute soul searching on my part since my return.*
> *I read the stories of you guys and your repeated trips (I think one guy has 59), and I begin to wonder, what, if anything keeps me here in the Estados Unitas?*
> *For every reason that I thought I had to remain here in the USA, I find more reasons not too.*
> *The obligations, commitments, and responsibilities that I thought were so important, pale in significance when I re–live in my memory the warm embrace, the shy smile, and the beauty of the "chica." The chica that are everywhere, and readily available, in that land of enchantment.*
> *I sat down and made a serious attempt at listing my reasons for staying home, alongside of my list for leaving.*
> *What is so surprising in reflection, was how readily I was able to xxx out those reasons on the "to stay" side.*
> *When I was finished, I came to the only conclusion that was possible for me.*
> *I AM GOING*[6]

McMonger is not a unique case. Three fourths of the sample at www.costaricaticas.com are either considering, are taking steps to move or have already settled in Costa Rica.[7]

Do you leave your life behind for a country that provides you with "smiles" and "warmth"? This seems odd, as mongers offer no specific plans of what life would be once in Costa Rica. Some who already settled in this country complain that once your addiction for the "*chicas*" diminishes life is rather boring and lonely. They argue that it is a passion that eventually fades away.

Prolijo, having already moved to Costa Rica and knowing the experiences of many other mongers gives a word of caution to McMonger. After all, he says, it is not the same to be on vacation than to permanently live in Costa Rica.

> *I don't mean to burst your bubble as I have a similar dream as yours –to move to CR as soon as I have the finances worked out. But I can't emphasize enough for you the importance of moving a lot slower. From what I understand you just*

finished your first trip. Teal has been going down 3–5X/yr for the past 15 years. VB and Sailfish are veterans of many trips as well. These guys have a much better idea of what CR is really all about than most of us. But did you notice that VB and Sailfish are renting and did not say anything about obtaining legal residency? I have spoken to many ex–pats living in CR and have researched about it over the web and in books and they all say the same thing –move slow. Nearly a universally recommendation is to try it on first. As DJ, pointed out what is fun for a week is not necessarily as much fun month after month. Sure going on vacation and banging lots of hookers is loads of fun, but you're not going to be on permanent vacation. Unless you are really rolling in dough, popping down $100/day on hookers like you do when you are on vacation is probably not part of your retirement budget. Besides you may find you tire of the tica mentality, or SJ traffic, CR bureaucracy, expensive automotive costs, and who knows what other aspect of CR that you failed to consider. Then again, maybe you won't. But you won't know for sure until you've been down there a while. Do what others recommend. [8]

Will Prolijo take this advice?

Notes

1. Kamala Kempadoo, *Sexing the Caribbean. Gender, Race and Sexual Labor,* London: Routledge, 2004, ebook, p. 465.
2. http://www.costaricaticas.com/phpbb2/viewtopic.php?t=1868
3. http://www.costaricaticas.com/phpbb2/viewtopic.php?t=638&highlight=poll
4. http://www.costaricaticas.com/phpbb2/viewtopic.php?t=2507
5. http://www.costaricaticas.com/phpbb2/viewtopic.php?t=2507
6. http://www.costaricaticas.com/phpbb2/viewtopic.php?t=1720
7. http://www.costaricaticas.com/phpbb2/viewtopic.php?t=1744&highlight=poll
8. http://www.costaricaticas.com/phpbb2/viewtopic.php?t=1720

14. Sex work becomes complicated

Ronnie Shaw in her study of American clients and Costa Rican sex workers recognized that sexual encounters are not exclusively for the "carnal act of sex:"

> *Interviewees professed a need for emotional fulfillment. A high school teacher from Michigan stated: "I've been married twice, divorced twice. I was tired of the bullshit back home...My former girlfriend was more interested in her career, pets, and even her mother more than me. My respondents never mentioned "true love;" however, their quest for emotional security and power within sexual transactions highlights the fact that prostitution may not be solely about the carnal act of sex.* [1]

Martin Opperman agrees with this view and thinks the search for love is the reason why prostitution in the West is no alternative for the American mongers:

> *Men also look for "love" in a customer–prostitute relationship– thus their "disappointment" in the commercial approach to prostitution in Western societies... perhaps this is the reason for some men to engage in sex tourism with planned sexual behavior with prostitutes in developing countries where their money supposedly can buy not only sex but also more tenderness on the side of prostitutes.* [2]

Mr. King Costa, a monger, jokingly proposed to build a chapel at Hotel Del Buey when he realized that many of his colleagues were involved in emotional relationships with sex workers.

> *As most of you know, my mind works in strange ways. I am totally shocked and blown away by how many mongers have GFs. Why not have a little wedding chapel in the Del Buey?*

> 1. *Great Image . . . Does the bride wear white? Imagine the bridesmaid's outfits purchased at Putas o Us.*
> 2. *Does the guest list include the numerous mongers that have been previous clients?*
> 3. *Does the groom get to select how many of the bridemaids he can include in their first after marriage sex session?*
> 4. *Will the band be the gut bucket guy, banjo guy, whistle guy and the other local musical talent?*
>
> *Will the bride and groom accept less than a cien for bridal gifts?* [3]

WilySP asks, "Whether in a wedding at this hotel do the groom or the bride as well as the guests seriously commit to a monogamous relationship?"

> *Of course I could see throwing condoms instead of rice. The bride would have a bottle of lub instead of flowers.*
> *The procession would have to weave through the gauntlet.*
> *I can see the happy couple at the rail the bride with the back of the dress conveniently raised allowing the guys in the audience to go a round before the ceremony was complete and the final "I DO" is said.*
> *Instead of a dollar dance there would be a 1,000 colonies blow job line up with the bride and all brides' maids.* [4]

Spanish Eyes, an online dating service, offers wives to American tourists. It promises to deliver feminine women.

> *Spanish Eyes Introductions specializes in the women who live in Costa Rica as they make the best wives and girlfriends. The women of Costa Rica are feminine not feminists. They are beautiful and sexy while retaining a degree of modesty and are respectful and supportive of their mates. We provide introductions to the most beautiful and sincere Ticas, as they like to refer to themselves. We are here to help you from the introduction to marriage and immigration.*[5]

Most online marriage agencies even display pictures of some of the weddings between North American men with Costa Rican ex–sex workers. The www.costaricachica.com website has an exclusive section for those who are looking for a girlfriend or a wife. [6]

Do people who are married and in love have a lesser chance of contracting the HIV virus?

Lupita's behavior is not encouraging. She tells us that she has to have sex on Saturday because "I am getting married on Sunday." We asked her whether she would use a condom with her date and she responded: "I see no point in using condoms since it is my farewell party from prostitution." Carmen is already married to an American doctor in the United States. She still practices sex work since "I need to save some money for any emergencies in the States." She doesn't use condoms either with her husband or with her regular clients. "What is the point?" she asks and continues, "Men like to have bareback sex with a bride to be."

Many American sex tourists become obsessed with knowing whether the sex worker is faithful to them. They even go so far as to ask other mongers if the women work at the hotels. Monger's desire for this kind of information has driven one monger to setting up a business to spy on sex workers: "Over the last several months, a number of mongers have become emotionally attached to those fine ladies in the BM. In fact, several of these guys want other mongers to "spy" on them and report back if these *chicas* are working at the BM." To satisfy this need for information King Costa has a solution to set up "a formal investigative group of mongers and named the business DEL BUEY MONGER SPY FOR HIRE. "Our mission and business plan is to provide all the spying you guys want and need for a fee."[7]

VegasBob agrees that there are many tourists who fall for the girls and the situation is rather desperate. Despite their asking around, mongers want to believe that "their relationship is different" and they "usually reject my help because it isn't what they want to hear." Despite the tendency to downplay the seriousness of this emotional involvement, the truth is that this "is far from humorous."[8]

Tourism scholar Erik Cohen, points to the same phenomenon in Thailand in an article entitled "*Transnational Marriage in Thailand: The Dynamics of Extreme Heterogamy.*"[9] Based on an exploratory study, the author examines the dynamics of transnational marriages between Western men (*farang*) and local Thai women. The author explains that the decision by foreign men to marry Thai women can be placed on a continuum that ranges from spontaneity to deliberation. In some cases the foreigner gets so infatuated with a Thai woman (often a prostitute) that he proposes marriage after only a week without checking the background of his future wife. The author notes that the majority of tourists who marry Thai women take them back to their countries of origin, which is also one of the principal motives that induce Thai women to marry foreigners. [10]

The risks taken when a relationship is taken to the category of friends or of love are high, as the following data indicates. We included in the 2000 Survey those relationships with men where money is not paid for sex. These men can be boyfriends, lovers, pimps, friends and husbands or anyone who has known the woman for sometime. 48% did not use condoms with their intimate partners. Among the respondents who currently have a partner, 86% do not use a condom, and among those who use it only 8% do it always. (Table 17)

Sex workers reported that they had control over the decision of whether or not to use the condom in these relationships. This means that they were willing to take risks with their partners. These partnerships based on trust and not on money turn to be the most dangerous for both actors with regard to HIV infection.

Sex workers reported that the main reason for not using condoms was when they were in intimate relationships (60%). (Table 18)

Marriage, therefore, could lead to unsafe sex and it does not preclude infecting others.

> *Hopefully this story will dissuade some of you from falling in love. There is a girl here that I have seen several times. She informed me that she met a Gringo recently, and "after knowing him for 7 days" she married him here in CR. In the same breath she tells me that he is back in Gringoland and when will I see her. She came to my house a couple of nights ago and it was sexo as usual.I asked her how long she had been married.She said "9 DAYS". Obviously no names and dates will be given here to protect the parties involved. Here in CR it is always better to rent than to buy.* [11]

Girlfriend fantasy experience

There are many grey areas between relationships that only engage in sex and those that involve love. Most mongers do not want to marry sex workers. On the other hand, the majority does not like to have causal sex. In between the two options, mongers have established a new type of relationship that is called Girlfriend Fantasy Experience (GFE). GFE is much more than being a regular partner and less so than being a husband. It has the intensity of a marriage and the shortness of a brief affair. It is not "real" but it does make people act as it was.

When sex tourists discuss in their forums what type of sexual tourist they are, the majority (55%) chooses the GFE option. Despite the different views of what the term means, it is associated with looking for some sort of intimate relationship with the sex worker. [12] Of this 55%, another Survey is taken to ask for further details on the *novia* relationships. According to the data, the relationships are established either with sex workers or not, either by residents or non–residents, with a professional or a non–professional sex worker. A "good" relationship is defined as "one that has lasted six months or more and did not end in the classical way of the girl making ever increasing and unreasonable demands for money." [13]

According to the Forum's sex expert, there are many men who would like to have a "*novia*." They want intimacy, passion and drama.

Guys who like "Novias"

1. *Intimate guy –A guy who arrives in CR, meets a gal he is attracted to, and simply likes the experience / illusion that he is getting closer– ie getting to know her. Kind of like a double life. Of course this can be dangerous, but if this is what they want . . . all the power to them.*
2. *Habit guy –A buy who likes a "constant". This is like going to your favorite restaurant. You know what you will be getting and like it. Sure you may order different items and appetizers on occasion, but you like that same favorite dish.*
3. *Novella guy –A guy who likes drama . . . and is kinda of a junkie. Usually likes the wild fluctuations in emotions and trives off of this.*
4. *The rescuer/Pretty woman guy –this guy likes to feel he is he ping to rescue a gal and show her a better life. Usually has plenty of disposable income that he would blow on something else (ie gambling)* [14]

Second houses

This is an institution that develops out of GFE and suggests a growing intensity in the relationship. It simply means that the customer sets up a house for the sex worker and sends her money. When he is in town, he acts as a lover and has a monopoly over the woman. When he leaves, she is "free" to go back to her old job. [15] As in regular relationships, men who set up a second house expect intimate and bareback sex. According to the polls in CostaRicatica.com, 30% of American tourists send money to the women.

Having a second house was common for men in 19th Century Latin America. Men would have a house for his wife and children and another for his lover and her children. Latin men abandoned this institution as it became too expensive to keep. Nowadays is the American male who is reviving the past and displaying one of the characteristics of Latin machismo.

Some tourists warn their colleagues of its dangers. One monger says that women usually ask for money and they promise, "They will be your loving fiancé and marry you!" This also happened to him:

> *Be very careful about this! I did this and was scammed but Good ! The woman that did this to me is still doing it to other men at this time also ! I am trying to find out who they are and warn and help them!*
> *I supported her for two years , until I discovered her scam . . . . She uses these men for there money and supports her "Tico" Boyfriend . . . If you are one of these men or know one . Please contact me ! I can put you in touch with the right people and lawyers so maybe we can stop her!* [16]

PacoLoco is aware that some mongers have second houses. Many of these men can be sharing the same woman who acts as a loving wife to each one. If the woman is infected, she might pass it to all her "husbands". Despite his awareness, Paco Loco still believes there could be an exception, which shows again how he also wants to delude himself.

> *I have a friend currently "paying" a chica not to work. He has been warned but is a big boy and it's his money. In my opinion it's stupid, will only turn out badly for him in the end and I wouldn't trust her as far as I could throw her, but then again she could be the one honest, sincere, ex–hooker in the country and they might live happily ever after.* [17]

King Costa attacks Astro for his naiveté in sending money to sex workers. He thinks it is a big business for the women and a terrible one for the men: "Let's assume she can convince 5 guys that they are special and convinces them to send them money on a regular basis in return for e mails, phone conversations and the promise of a great time when they return." If each sends her $300 a month, "She now has a residual income of $1,500 to do virtually nothing and if you add sex work, she makes double money." "What is the advantage for the Gringo," he asks: "Not much really, usually takes no more than 5 minutes to find another one. Sometimes 10 if you are a little slow or drunk." And the disadvantage?"

1. *Now you cannot monger without all of her phuckin friends ratting you out. Everytime she need extra money she is gonna hit you up.*
2. *You have to listen to all her problems.*
3. *She might get pregnant.*

Once King Costa summarizes all these stories, he suggests to his fellow mongers: "NO NOVIA RULE..." [18]

Others such as Goetzvonberlishingen think that sex workers can make more money without having to set up emotional relationships and that when they do; they sabotage their arrangements by demanding too much financially.

> *Once a chica establishes a novio relationship with her gringo, why do they insist on pressing the monetary demands exponentially to the point of termination of the relationship? ...*
> *They kill the golden goose and then have to start the hunt and the breakin all over again. How stupid. It would be much smarter and more productive to keep the demands small and reasonable and go for the long term and cultivate guys they can enjoy anyway.*
> *So that's the question, why do chicas insist on getting more and more ridiculous with their requests for money until we blow them off instead of making their*

pursuit easier with pleasant reasonable relationships. [19]

Flander believes the women will demand more money whether there is a financial crisis or not. He was dating a woman twenty years younger than him. She used to work in the States and had purchased a car and a home in Costa Rica. Nevertheless, when he visited her "everytime im (sic) in sjo there is a crisis of some sort in her personal life that requires money. will not go into detail but some of them are down right inventive and very clever. ..i have come to the conclusion that all ticas, regardless of age, socio economic status whatever are born to the hustle. no matter that they dont need the money, its a game to get it from any gringo they find and the more the better.." [20]

Witling, finally, suggests other mongers to put themselves in the women's shoes.

My opinion and of course there are exceptions to everything:

1. *Most of the full–time working girls are not educated.*
2. *They see things in black and white (and green).*
3. *Their future visions only consist of the next score except for their fantasies. I've seen girls talking about "how much they got" for a 1 hour tryst.*
4. *As King Costa mentioned, they think all Gringos are rich, and we are, compared to them. Afterall, don't we fly to Costa Rica and blow hundreds of dollars 2 or 3 (or more) times a year?*
5. *Guys come and go, the only constants for these girls are their niños and their families and the need to make money. They know there are no guarantees so they get what they can before it runs out. Also consider many of these girls have, somewhere in their past, been abused or at least taken advantage of by a male. It might have been an abusive father, a local "novio" or a customer, but most do have scars. Their perspective on men, especially customers, has jaded them somewhat.*

*Think of it like this, you grew up poor, you quit school at the age of 14, you have a Ch*ld to feed, suddenly someone tells you that they will pay you more than you've ever earned in you life just for doing something you used to do for free. Suddenly you think you've hit the lottery and it will never run out.* [21]

The institution of a second house is another avenue to HIV infection. It involves the sex worker and her client, her intimate partner and her client's and any other sexual partner that either one may have. Prolijo's wife might feel quite safe back in Florida with regard to HIV infection. Paco Loco' s sexual partner, who works at Walmart in Kentucky, might never feel to be a part of a HIV group risk. But the stark truth is that both women are having unsafe sex with partners who are among the most vulnerable to get AIDS. A "*novia*" is not necessarily the woman you have a second house with. She might be someone you date more than once. Clients admit not using condoms with their "novias": "I hate condoms. I hate them, I really do, but with boinking (sic), I wear one, with the exception of a couple of my novias."[22]

To study the relationship between intimacy and sex, we included in the 2000 Survey those relationships with men where money is not paid for sex. These men can be boyfriends, lovers, pimps, friends and husbands or anyone who has known the woman for sometime.

48% of the sex workers did not use condoms with their intimate relationships. (Table 18). Nevertheless, among the respondents who currently have a partner, 86% do not use a condom, and among those who use it only 8% do it always. Sex workers reported that they had control over the decision of whether or not to use the condom in these relationships. This means that they express trust with the practice of taking risks with partners. These partnerships based on trust and not on money turn to be the most dangerous for both actors with regard to HIV infection. Sex workers reported that the main reason for not using condoms was when they were in relationships (60%). (Table 18)

We asked María to tell us what sort of man is the one she is intimate with. She responds that it is a man who is a friend of hers. We then ask her to tell us what does it take to become a friend. She thinks that it takes time. "A friend is someone who I know for a while"- she answers. "How long is the minimum you need to know someone?" We inquired. "At least a week"- she indicates. "Then we can say that if you meet someone on Monday for sex and he comes next week for another session, he is already a friend?" She waits for a minute and responds positively. "Do you use condoms with friends?"- We insist. "With some I do and with others I don't"- she responds. "How about with a "*novio*" or a lover?"-We wanted to know. "With people I am in love with I don't use condoms"- she says. "Who are you in love with?"-We insisted. "Those men who are good to me"- is her response. "Are these men the ones who send you money, bring you gifts and see you more regularly?"- We inquired. "Yes, a friend is a person that cares for you"-She states. "Do Americans can be considered your friends and lovers?" We asked. "I only consider American men to be serious enough for that"–she responds.

Given Marías' view of friendship, it is to be expected she would not use regularly condoms with regular partners (those who come more than once), "*novios*", lovers or husbands.

"When you are in love –she concludes– one does not know what a fool you can be."

Notes

1. Ronnie Shaw, *Fantasy Voyages: An Exploration of White Males' Participation in the Costa Rican Sex Tourism Industry* [90] The Berkeley McNair Research Journal, p.3
2. Martin Opperman, "Introduction" in Opperman, *Sex Tourism and Prostitution: Aspects of Leisure, Recreation and Work,* edited by Martin Opperman, 1–19. New York: Cognizant Communication Corporation. 1998, 157
3. http://www.costaricaticas.com/phpbb2/viewtopic.php?t=3909
4. http://www.costaricaticas.com/phpbb2/viewtopic.php?t=3909
5. http://www.spanisheyes.com
6. Ronnie Shaw, *Fantasy Voyages: An Exploration of White Males' Participation in the Costa Rican Sex Tourism Industry* [90] The Berkeley McNair Research Journal, 2004.
7. http://www.costaricaticas.com/phpbb2/viewtopic.php?t=3669
8. http://www.costaricaticas.com/phpbb2/viewtopic.php?t=3669
9. Thomas B. Bawer and Bob McKercher, *Sex and Tourism Journeys of Romance, Love, and Lust,* Editors The Haworth Hospitality Press®An Imprint of The Haworth Press, Inc. New York • London • Oxford, 2003, p.57.
10. Thomas B. Bawer and Bob McKercher, *Sex and Tourism Journeys of Romance, Love, and Lust,* Editors The Haworth Hospitality Press®An Imprint of The Haworth Press, Inc. New York • London • Oxford, 2003, p.57.
11. http://www.costaricaticas.com/phpbb2/viewtopic.php?
12. http://www.costaricaticas.com/phpbb2/viewtopic.php?t=2934&highlight=poll
13. http://www.costaricaticas.com/phpbb2/viewtopic.php?t=3888
14. http://www.costaricaticas.com/phpbb2/viewtopic.php?t=3401
15. http://www.costaricaticas.com/phpbb2/viewtopic.php?t=3401
16. http://www.costaricaticas.com/phpbb2/viewtopic.php?t=3401
17. http://www.costaricaticas.com/phpbb2/viewtopic.php?t=3401
18. http://www.costaricaticas.com/phpbb2/viewtopic.php?t=3401
19. http://www.costaricaticas.com/phpbb2/viewtopic.php?t=3401
20. http://www.costaricaticas.com/phpbb2/viewtopic.php?t=3401
21. http://www.costaricaticas.com/phpbb2/viewtopic.php?t=2610
22. http://www.costaricaticas.com/phpbb2/viewtopic.php?t=939&postdays=0&pos-torder=asc&start=15

15. Ethics

Both mongers and sex workers feel very strongly on what is right and wrong. The men rationalize prostitution mostly on socio biological grounds. GetRhythm, for example, tells his views to an American friend he met in Costa Rica. They went on a date and had a couple of drinks together and then he decided to "let the cat of the bag concerning the types of massages I'd had on my recent trip to Costa Rica." The woman did not like his sharing of this information and told him she felt sad for the poor women who "are forced by their economic situations to engage in sex for pay. She went on to say that if these girls lived in a society where they had better opportunities, then this type of thing wouldn't exist." [1] GetRhythm did not like her response and gave her a piece of his mind on this topic:

> *I say balderdash! Prostitution has existed throughout history for one basic reason –there is a demand for it. Many women don't seem to understand that men are simply wired differently. Because of our different ancestral roles, we require sex more often and prefer to have it with a greater variety of partners. Of course, this doesn't rule out the possibility of finding satisfaction in a loving monogamous relationship, but nevertheless, the temptation will always be there. Don't know if I'll be having dinner again with my friend anytime soon, but no matter –my next trip to CR isn't far in the future.* [2]

Most mongers think that because men have a genetic make–up to spread their seeds, they need to have sex with lots of women. This biological need explains why women back home cannot satisfy the men's more "promiscuous" tendencies. Men's ability to have sex with multiple partners without emotional involvement can also be explained by gender. Feminist theory, for example, promotes a view of sex as culturally–constructed where men are trained, not born, to enjoy multiple partners and paid–sex. Nevertheless, mongers do not like this framework as it calls for personal responsibility to modify sexual conditioning and for being respectful toward woman's sexuality. It is much easier for them to explain their sexual behavior on the basis of genes, hormones or brain "wires," whatever that means.

The men are aware that prostitution is not ethically acceptable to the majority of the population. Ruffunutz recommends to a monger who is planning to take his son to monger along with him in Costa Rica, that this might not be a good idea: "I want to be clear on what I am saying, I am not saying that mongering is BAD, but you really don't know if your son may in fact think it is, and you being the one exposing him to this lifestyle will forever create an association between you, the father, and mongering in his head. . . if he so happens to think that it's wrong in any way, it may change your relationship and his opinion of you for the worst. Not to mention the fact that you will burden him with the knowledge of your infidelity to his mother, which puts him in a very bad situation, as he will be torn between keeping the secret and betraying his mom or revealing what he knows and betraying you, either way he loses . . . not a fun place to be."[3]

Mongers see prostitution in terms of needs and rights. One has a right to pursue something that is lacking –a need– and the other has the right to sell it. In a market economy, sex is not seen more different than any other services. When it does, as in the United States, it is because of prudishness and hypocrisy. The sex tourists admire Costa Rica where prostitution is legal.

The right to pay for sex should be framed in a consumer's morality. According to this perspective, the monger is a client who buys a product and hence is entitled to receive a good service. This means that the women who sell sexual services must do it professionally and without taking advantage of the customer.

Mongers are aware that women sell their bodies because of a lack of job skills, because of poverty or to fulfill a need for goods that are scant in third world countries: "I suppose if it wasn't for the 'third world' countries –those far less fortunate than us, we wouldn't find the inexpensive, available material for the exercise of our passionate hobby of whore–mongering. The misfortune of these societies provides the economic basis for our affordable pleasure." Nevertheless, to buy their services is moral –they say– because prostitution allows the poor women to improve their lot and that of their families: "As a 'monger', I support these girls. Without me and people like me, they would starve. Luckily, there is no shortage of men anywhere in the world who are looking for the services they provide."

Sex tourists do not think they can do much to change economic handicaps: "Would I change that if I could? You bet. Do I have the power? No way. I learned a long time ago, I can't change the world; I can only try in my small ways to make it a better place by my actions and behavior." According to him, there is no reason to feel guilty: "No, I do not apologize for being a monger...I will give them money for the crises that they always seem to have –if I have seen them several times and enjoy their company, I am willing to do that. I never promise what I can't or won't deliver. No promise of marriage, no promise of 'living with me in California' and no promise that I will buy or rent a place in TJ or Rosarita that they can live in and 'keep up' for me. That would be more than unfair, it would be cruel because it won't happen." "Likewise, I would not ask them for exclusivity. That would not be economically feasible, emotionally fair or reasonable to expect."[4]

Fr. Lust believes that by paying for sex he is fighting famine and destitution. He does not want to marry the woman or to bring her home, but he feels nonetheless that he is doing something positive.

Goal gets "annoyed" when other mongers negatively judge sex workers for their work. He is convinced Costa Rican sex workers do it to support their children and that contrary to what happens in the United States, they do not spend the money on drugs. Since sex money feeds kids, it is good money. This monger thinks that he is no different than any well–meaning organization such as UNICEF that helps third world kids.[5]

Men see this transaction as a sort of investment in the social development of the sex workers, something similar to the loans rich governments provide to the underdeveloped world. It is like building a country's infrastructure (education, health, food). They reason that thanks to them these women have a chance to improve their lives and their standard of living. Sex money should be therefore seen as a kind of loan that is up to the woman to put to good use. Mexpat says that "My thought was that once a *chica* has made the decision to sell her ass for money in the BM . . . THEN . . . if she continued to live in poverty, it would be her own fault. In the BM environment it seems to me certainly possible for any reasonably attractive *chica* who dedicates herself to "*la vida facìl*" to make a very good living if she applies herself."[6]

But as any major bank that lends money to the third world, mongers find it frustrating when the women do not appreciate this investment and give back a lousy service in return.

Price is a major ethical concern. The money issue is –as we have seen before– complicated. First of all, there is not a set price on sex. "What is fair to pay?" –a monger asks. Some argue that Costa Rican women should not charge, as much as prostitutes in the United States whose tag is $300 an hour. They reason that since the cost of living is much lower in the third world, sex workers should charge less for their services.

The problem is that mongers do not know what the "lowest" rate should be and many admit to know fellow–mongers who easily pay $200 an hour. In order to prevent prices from rising, mongers strategize. The first thing they do is to keep Costa Rica to themselves to avoid a flood of sex tourists that would drive the rates up. Secondly, they agree among themselves to pay no more than 100 bucks an hour. This "*no cien*" policy is enforced through mutual solidarity and advices in the sex forums.

Some of the tactics seem to be the tools of a Socialist economy than a capitalist one. Don Gordo, for example, recommends lowering prices through economic starvation. He tells his friends to wait until the sex worker is desperate: When women find they might go home alone, they will drop the prices. Vegas Bob tells other mongers to hide their willingness to buy: "If you don't look horny, you have more leverage"- he writes. Uncle Sam, as a new Columbus, suggests to others to exchange American trinkets for sex. "Sex workers think American chocolates are really expensive. Give them some and ask for a discount"- he says. Don Giovanni uses the poor's strategy to inspire pit: act as a therapist and listen to the sex worker's sad stories in exchange for halving her asking price. King Costa, finally, suggests going for the not–so–attractive sex worker to get a better price: "In general, the hotter looking the *chica* is, the more likely she will put you on the clock. In many cases, *sexo* is very mechanical. *Chicas* with a few flaws such as age, weight, face issues or simply a lack of experience in many cases will provide you with a better experience simply because they are not in the highest demand."[7]

According to mongers, sex workers should be paid according to their good looks. Top sex workers, rated at 10, can charge more for the hour. Younger prostitutes are entitled to ask for more and those who are adolescents can get the most dollars. If the woman provides an excellent sexual performance, which includes oral sex, she might be entitled to top money. The same goes for time. A whole night should be more expensive than a single hour; an entire weekend or month more than a day. Nevertheless, when the deal includes more than one day, the woman has to provide sex anytime and anywhere. Mongers make their own calculations to get the price of each sexual act right. McMonger, for example, tells other mongers that if they pay $700 a week and have sex three times a day, the rate for each sex act has come down to $33, a real bargain. Papa Nut is not so sure. He responds to McMonger that he forgets to include food, Viagra and entertainment. These items must be added up to the costs. According to Papa Nut, the price is therefore closer to $40 per sex act.[8]

Price bargaining is not that common in the States. Mongers admit that they would not dream of asking for lower prices from American prostitutes. Nevertheless, as people in Latin America try to overcharge the tourist, they believe it is fair that the tourist fights back. So much they haggle that VegasBob thinks that mongers have gone overboard. First of all, he admits to agree with the mantra of "No Cien Policy" to some of the sex workers like "the "Colombianas with the silicone tetas who usually spend even less than an hour for the cien." Nevertheless, some mongers have made this advice into a general policy and make the mistake of excluding "chicas who are the best GFE experiences."[9]

As part of the mongers' morality, customers should not be imposed extra payments. Romulus finds unethical that girls negotiate downstairs a price and ask for another upstairs: "She is quite attractive and has full lips and shoulder length black hair. She will accept whatever price you agree upon downstairs and when you get to the room she will ask for $100 and to pay up front. Watch out for her and warn everyone else you can about her!"[10]

Sex workers are not supposed to ask for money for transportation or communication. It is not up to the customer to pay for their cell phones. They should not expect the customer to buy them gifts either, with the exception of those in "*novia*" relationships. It is not moral to ask for money for children, relatives, groceries or clothes. More importantly, sex workers should not steal. According to mongers those who do steal should be prosecuted and expelled from the sex industry. Some customers feel so betrayed that they propose to have their photos taken and to expose them as thieves in the Internet. The forums have warnings on many *chicas* who steal and so does the Hotel Del Buey that keeps a file on them. Administrator 1 gives the 10 moral commandments for sex mongers:

> *Thou shall not pay any Chica cien for 1 hour!*
> *Thou shall not send money to a Tica from the US!*
> *Thou shall always backup a CRT member by being an on–call wingman!*
> *Thou shall freely help other CRT mongers in need of advice!*
> *Thou shall always act like a gentlemen and not ruin the CRT Name!*
> *A) Thou shall not drink too much and behave like an ugly American!*
> *B) Be respectful of the ladies, but also the "civilian" tourists and hotel staff.*
> *C) Respect other members and chicas anonymity, get permission before posting pics.*
> *D) Great service? Give a tip!*
> *E) Be aware and keep valuables locked up.*
> *Thou shall not ever share the secrets of CRT or give Ticas access to pictures!*
> *Thou shall not a GFE threaten or take over your life!*
> *Thou shall not ever pay upfront!*
> *Thou shall not be so intoxicated as to become an easy victim!*[11]

One of the major monger's complaints is the abuse of time. If the woman sells herself by the hour, it is expected that she stays for the entire sixty minutes.

Mongers feel ripped off when they finish in a few minutes and the sex worker decides the session is over. In www.costaricaTicas.com, a poll shows that most mongers do not want their sexual encounters to be less than an hour. [12]

What is the preferred length of your sexual encounters?		
I prefer quickies, in and out in under 1 hour.	5%	[4]
An hour or two is good for me.	47%	[33]
I like a "date". Maybe dinner/dancing then sex.	15%	[11]
I like all–nighters with something in the morning, too.	21%	[15]
I'll hit it as hard as I can for as long as I can.	10%	[7]
	Total Votes:	70 [13]

As a customer, the client has the right to request the woman to stay either for more sex, a massage or a simple conversation. Goal is of the idea that he is entitled to come as many times as possible in sixty minutes and gets annoyed when the sex worker asks for more money. Nevertheless, when the situation is reversed and the monger cannot ejaculate within the hour, he feels exploited if the sex worker decides to leave.

A poor service is one that is done without passion and love for your work. As any other business, prostitution should be done with gusto. If the woman does it with lack of interest, she is being unethical since she fails to come up with the goods. Mongers consider immoral to pay one hundred dollars for those who are "professional": "Hopefully we all know that the "*no cien*" is for the hardcore *putas* who want to go give you a quickie rubber Phuck with no contact, no passion, no time, as soon as they can get your drunken ass to C*m or pass out and flee with your money." [14]

Sexual practices must be diverse. Sexual tourists expect to own the woman's body for the time agreed. This means that the sex worker should be willing to do all that is asked of her. When a woman refuses to engage in French kissing, oral sex or anal sex she is perceived as dishonest. She may charge more for painful or difficult practices yet she should not reject it outright.

A major moral flaw is to fake, to simulate and to lie. Mongers believe the woman should not fake the orgasm. They believe she should enjoy the sex even though she is getting paid for it. Besides, most think they have the "proper equipment" to satisfy women.. In the first place, as we saw in former chapters, they think they are better lovers and friends than Latino men. Secondly, they think that they have larger genitals.

Mongers make fun of sex workers for trying to make them believe that they are well endowed. Vegas Bob laughs at the "*chicas* extoling the virtue of my 'incredible' thing with comments such as Papi Papi you have a big D*ck." He says, on the one hand, that "you'd think that all we guys should be making movies" and that "The *chicas* in CR all seem to say that anything over an inch and a half belongs in a museum." [15] In a poll, 65% of the customers say that sex workers do not care about size and prefer smaller organs. [16]

Once the mongers agree that there is nothing unusual about their sexual endowment, they start revisiting their conclusions and delude themselves with the theory that perhaps sex workers are not fooling them after all. VegasBob doubts his own hypothesis. He tells his readers that he "took a legitimate 18 year old first timer out of the DB and to my house." He found out that the girl "is a virgin," something doubtful for a woman who is found at Del Buey. He adds that the girl was "really astonished" to discover his penis size: "As we were playing on the couch we disrobed each other. She put her hand around my manhood and said innocently 'is this normal?' I'll be damned if she didn't earn a *propina (tip)* right there." [17]

Other mongers agree with VegasBob that they are indeed well endowed: Dick67 says "These guys are real mongers with the necessary equipment to satisfy the chicas in demand. I'm proud of my well hung status......must have gotten it from grand dad." [18] Astroglide agrees with Vegas Bob and reports that sex workers are impressed by his penis size. He thought to be "average" before going to Costa Rica. But once he went to his bedroom with Cristal and Joelly, the former sex worker "was bragging to her friend Joelly about me..." When they finally took their clothes off, "she showed Joelly the merchandise, and she seemed impressed." He is now "sure" that the women were not joking and if anyone "has any doubts" Astroglide informs VegasBob that he uses Trojan Magnum condoms since the "regular condoms fit too tight and hurt me." [19]

According to monger's morale, the woman as a provider must ensure that her "equipment" is clean and in good shape. Mongers like Costa Rican women because they are extremely clean and shower frequently. They give laudatory remarks because they take care that their sexual organs do not smell and that this makes it easier for them to practice vaginal oral sex. Sluthog wants to know, for example, whether it is safe to do it: "Although I have been very tempted on occasion to DATY on some beautiful pro or semi–pro I just haven't been able to get past the fact of who has been there before me! Time to fess up; who dares to really and truly "lick the whisker biscuit"? [20] Piroca responds that he's done it and that the girls are so clean no one had ever guessed what they had done before: "I did last week to a REALLY Hot young girl that tasted Great and acted like no one had ever done that to her before (that's Good!!). And I DO NOT have any cold sores!!!" [21]

They disapprove of some foreign sex workers who are not so clean. In such cases, they feel entitled to ask for a replacement and not to pay for the session.

Sex tourists expect the women to be tested. It is their responsibility to know whether they are HIV infected or not. Mongers constantly ask other mongers whether they know if the sex workers get their medical check–ups. As customers they do not seem to have the same concerns. They do not expect to be tested to ensure they will not infect the women.

As customers, mongers believe they also have some moral responsibilities.

It is ethical to respect the woman's privacy. Sexual tourists should not reveal the woman's identity. Mongers are aware that posting the woman's picture in Internet is a violation of her rights and a threat to her security. Most of them do not respect this rule, but they have moral concerns for breaking it.

Sex tourists also feel responsible for reckless behavior. If the woman gets pregnant, for example, they feel that is their responsibility to provide for her. They would make sure that she gets a DNA test to prove that the child is his, but it would not be ethical to walk away. If she gets sick because of drugs or intoxication while in their company, mongers feel they should take her to a private clinic or hospital. Despite these moral guidelines, the sex forums are filled with posts of stories of mongers who fled from these situations. Sex tourists are aware that Costa Rican paternity laws are strict and that a man who fails to take a DNA test is legally assumed to be a father and is responsible for child support. According to some mongers, the best alternative to avoid the law and the situation "is to take the first plane out of the country."

Mongers have more responsibilities with novias. This includes buying them presents, paying for clothes, taking them out, inviting them to vacations, and in some cases, providing allowances, loans and money for the children's tuition.

Money is for Astroglide the trick that does the magic to turn a prostitute into a friend: "But for this investment, every time . . . I have seen the girl change right before my eyes."

Astroglide says that if he pays $100, sex gets much better: "In the case of Katherine, she went from giving me 75% to 150% in bed." For only $25 extra, he says, "She goes from seeing me as a customer to a friend."[22] He recognizes that "it might be true that I spend too much money on them," but it is worth the price. He suggests that not only pays to pay more for sex, but to provide sex workers with unsolicited gifts: "As for Keren, the sweetheart that took me to the airport, she was shocked that I offered her money and tried not to accept it until I insisted."[23]

Gringotim is aware that the gifts often end up in someone else's hands: "Many times I've given CD players, CDs, and various other gifts to *chicas*. When I see them on subsequent trips, many times they've told me that they no longer have the gift(s)...they were stolen!" Despite of this, he sincerely believes the presents were welcomed: "Oh well, at least they enjoyed the gifts a little while, and I know they were always appreciated,"[24]

They expect the woman to be faithful. If the woman is not exclusive when the monger is gone, she must be when he spends his time in Costa Rica. If the woman is faithful, she in entitled to gain more money. Nevertheless, one thing is to ask for money once, and another to do it more than once. John, a monger, "admitted to me that he sent $200 bucks via Western Union on two occasions . . . and he now regrets it." According to him, "The problem is simple . . . if you continue to communicate with them . . . either by phone or e–mail, they will eventually ask for help." But since these women "live in near poverty," they will try to squeeze as much as possible from them. John admits that he "can't blame them" since "They do not know what is appropriate to ask for." The solution, for him, should be simple: "I just say . . . no gracias. I can't do that. They back off."[25]

Unless the American tourist marries the sex worker, she should not expect to be taken to the United States or to share the man's life back home. Mongers are adamant that the "*noviazgo*" ends at the airport and that they do not want to mix their "real" life in the States with the one in Costa Rica. In a small number of cases, when they do take the sex workers to the United States, they are required to be faithful wives and companions.

Sex workers have a moral system of their own. Contrary to the monger's ethics that is based on customers' rights and investments in third world development, women have a religious family morality to explain and rationalize their behavior. This means it is ethical to engage in prostitution to help your children and next to kin to survive and improve their lives. When your choices are made for the family's survival, your sins are forgiven. Therefore, every act is judged according to how it affects the family. Nancy tells us "Jesus forgives me because He knows that I am doing it for my family."

The women might or might not help their families or they might or might not be in a desperate economic situation, but either way their rationale is that they practice prostitution to help others. The women usually consider prostitution to be sinful and absolution comes by practicing altruistic acts.

María believes that what she is doing is wrong. She goes to church often and when asked what she prays for, she responds that "I ask Jesus Christ to take me away from this life." María expects that Jesus will give her a sign to leave. The idea that powerful forces have control over people's decisions is not foreign to sexual minorities who lack traditional forms of power. But if María is still in prostitution is because "Jesus does not want me to leave yet. He knows when will the right time will be."

Most sex workers have children to support. They obtain absolution from local Costa Rican friends who also hold the view that poverty excuses immoral behavior. Carlos, a taxi driver, thinks that sex workers will be forgiven by a loving God who understands that poor people must survive. The same is shared by José, a bartender at the hotel El Duende: "Sex workers work for their families and what they do is hard work. I respect them for being so sacrificial."

The women explain other unlawful behavior in terms of a Robinhood morality. If they steal from tourists is to share their wealth with the poor. Ana admitted that she often gets into the man's wallet to make extra money. When we asked her whether she thought it was right to do so, she responded that it was not wrong to do it since she gave the money to poorer people in her neighborhood. "I help doña Carmen, a beggar with these extras"- she argues. Inés thinks that trying to get as much as possible from her customers is fair because "these men have lots of money and they waste their money on women anyhow." Glenda rationalizes her stealing for her jealousy: "I rip them off so they cannot buy more women."

It is important for the women to divide sex work from love. Therefore, to hold the belief that it is moral to do sex work for economic reasons then it is crucial that the economic sphere remains apart from the emotional dimension. This translates to sex with customers should no be fun. This means that sex workers do certain things with clients and others with lovers and friends. French kissing, oral and anal sex are reserved for intimate relationships, so is vaginal sex without a condom. When these practices are combined with both customers and lovers, sex workers fear of their reputations. Lucy, for example, says she is a decent whore since she does not give blowjobs. Esther says she is good because she never practices anal sex as some of those "dirty crack whores from the street."

As the division between work and love is made by sex workers, time is a contested territory. Most women want to finish the sexual encounter with their clients as fast as possible. It is ethical to rush the man to come since "I do it without feeling anything. The fastest the better", says Fancy. Simulation in this regard has contradictory moral values. On the one hand, pretending to have an orgasm helps rush the customer to have his; on the other, it suggests the woman is having sexual pleasure, a feeling she should not be having.

Sex workers want money and the more the merrier. Wanting money and demanding lots of it is a sign you do sex only for economic reasons. There are moral limits to making money though. For sex workers, it becomes morally unsound when you risk your life for extra bucks. "I use a condom because I cannot afford to get HIV and make my children orphans," reports Sarita. Lupe also thinks that the desire for money must stop at the point the sex worker life becomes at risk. "I think some girls are so sick they do anything for money, including bareback sex. They are morally sick because they don't think of their kids."

Sex workers see prostitution income as "sinful money" that should be spent as soon as possible. As any drug smuggler would, sex workers have ethical problems with regard to how they made the money. It is usually seen as "dirty" and "immoral" money. One way to deal with the guilt is to spend it as quickly as possible. "I hate the 100 dollar bills. It is so obvious that I have them because of what I do. As soon as I get them, I want to buy something else, any object that is not money anymore"- reveals Karina. In other circumstances, spending money is a sort of laundering to avoid being asked for loans. Lupita buys clothes because she knows that if her mother sees the money, she will ask for a loan.

> *What you hate about the Ticas is also what you love about them. Most of us work save and invest. Save some, spend some. For them . . . it seems that the truly live for the moment. If they work tonight and make $100, well, then tomorrow they spend the $100. They may pay the rent, get some food, pay the babysitter, buy some clothes . . . but then they are broke again and back to the well they come for more "water".*[26]

Both mongers and sex workers care about ethics. Nevertheless, their frameworks are quite different. Clients believe that health prevention is part of a customer's right and that sex workers should check themselves periodically. On the other hand, sex workers think health prevention is a family responsibility. The woman who gets infected is putting other relatives or her children at risk. Interestingly enough, both the sex workers and the sexual clients seem to be oblivious of one another. Mongers do not assume any responsibility for protecting sex workers and the latter also do not consider their customer's health to be of moral obligation.

Liminal people have strong moral stands but they also assume risk is inherent in their lifestyles. The chat rooms are filled with warnings on STIs but also with attacks to those who are too concerned on being infected. "If you want to live until you are one hundred, perhaps you should not be mongering", says McMonger.

Sex workers also advice each other about many of the risks they face, from violence to blackmail to AIDS. But they also say "*De algo hay que morirse*" (You will die sooner or later).

Notes

1. http://www.costaricaticas.com/phpBB2/viewtopic.php?t=4230
2. http://www.costaricaticas.com/phpBB2/viewtopic.php?t=4230
3. http://www.costaricaticas.com/phpbb2/viewtopic.php?t=4321
4. http://www.costaricaticas.com/phpbb2/viewtopic.php?t=97
5. http://www.costaricaticas.com/phpbb2/viewtopic.php?t=97
6. http://www.costaricaticas.com/phpbb2/viewtopic.php?t=82&postdays=0&pos-torder=asc&highlight=sending+money&start=15

7. http://www.costaricaticas.com/phpBB2/viewtopic.php?t=4608
8. http://www.costaricaticas.com/phpBB2/viewtopic.php?t=4608
9. http://www.costaricaticas.com/phpbb2/viewtopic.php?t=4312
10. http://www.costaricaticas.com/phpbb2/viewtopic.php?t=3442
11. http://www.costaricaticas.com/phpbb2/viewtopic.php?t=4363
12. http://www.costaricaticas.com/phpBB2/viewtopic.php?t=4627
13. http://www.costaricaticas.com/phpBB2/viewtopic.php?t=4627
14. http://www.costaricaticas.com/phpbb2/viewtopic.php?t=4312
15. http://www.costaricaticas.com/phpbb2/viewtopic.php?t=3503
16. http://www.costaricaticas.com/phpbb2/viewtopic.php?t=3503
17. http://www.costaricaticas.com/phpbb2/viewtopic.php?t=3503
18. http://www.costaricaticas.com/phpbb2/viewtopic.php?t=3503
19. http://www.costaricaticas.com/phpbb2/viewtopic.php?t=3503
20. http://www.costaricaticas.com/phpbb2/viewtopic.php?t=3503
21. http://www.costaricaticas.com/phpbb2/viewtopic.php?t=4335
22. http://www.costaricaticas.com/phpbb2/viewtopic.php?t=82
23. http://www.costaricaticas.com/phpbb2/viewtopic.php?t=82
24. http://www.costaricaticas.com/phpbb2/viewtopic.php?t=82&postdays=0&postorder=asc&highlight=sending+money&start=15
25. http://www.costaricaticas.com/phpbb2/viewtopic.php?t=3503
26. http://www.costaricaticas.com/phpBB2/viewtopic.php?t=4465

16. HIV

In 1990, The Costa Rican AIDS' Survey showed that Costa Ricans were aware of HIV and its prevention, but they nevertheless practiced unsafe sex. [1] With regard to sex workers, our 1997 and the 2000 Surveys provide similar data. Sex workers, for example, knew what the best strategies were to avoid infection. When asked what recommendations they would make to a friend to prevent HIV (Table 25), more than 95% of the women stated that they would suggest her to use condoms with regular or causal partners. 90% also would advice her to refrain from anal sex. They also indicated in large percentages (Table 26) to have followed these same safe sex techniques. The women were aware that alcohol and drug consumption were dangerous to prevention and should be avoided. However, as we have seen before, these same respondents do not apply these rules to their lovers or partners. Sex workers recommended to others to use condoms, but more than half admitted not using them with regular clients and partners.

Mongers are no different in this behavior. The sex forums are filled with advice like "mongers, mongers wrap your dongues" that as we have seen in this study, are not heeded most of the time. The sex tourists are more knowledgeable than sex workers on the risks involved in unsafe sex. Some of them are so up–to–date that their posts indicate they are written by doctors and other health practitioners. Their recommendations on safe sex are no less accurate than those made by the experts in the field. Nevertheless, the same men who provide estimates of the risks involved in brushing your teeth prior to engaging in oral sex or in French kissing after having a root canal are also causally admitting having bareback sex with a "*novia*", who happens to be a professional prostitute.

The problem is not knowledge or lack thereof. It is attitudes, beliefs and psychological mechanisms such as denial or wishful thinking that lead people to slip with regard to HIV prevention. [2] We have seen that intimacy issues, alcohol consumption and money are the main culprits.

During our two RAPS and from the sex forums we asked sex workers and mongers to provide us with some innovative ideas to do HIV prevention. After all, they are the experts in the field and they know better than anyone else, including health experts, what is that they need to protect themselves.

Female condom

Sex workers, such as María, manifested a strong interest in using the female condom. Most of them suggested this would be a great opportunity to empower themselves. Nevertheless, they were not familiar with the product and wanted to learn more about it. In a study made with Family Health International (A study on the acceptability of the female condom by low class sex workers) women indicated their willingness to use it. Once they tried it, they reported that many clients did not even notice they had it on. [3] (Table 20) They thought the female condom made safe sex much easier for them and that it provided them with more security. This data suggests it is more viable to promote the female condom among sex workers who cater to tourists than those that work in the lower–income sector since they have the available income to afford the product, which is twenty times more expensive than the male condom.

The female condom is important because women are biologically more vulnerable to transmission from an infected partner than men are. More important, economic, social, and cultural disempowerment means that the current HIV prevention strategies of abstinence, monogamy, condom use, fewer partners, and treatment of sexually transmitted infections (STI's) are not feasible for many women, since they often lack the ability to negotiate safe sex. [4] Therefore, there is an urgent need for HIV prevention strategies that give women greater control to protect their bodies. The female condom is the only female–controlled safe–sex method available. While this method is effective and relatively well accepted by women; costs, men's negative attitudes, its contraceptive properties, and practical aspects of its use limit its usefulness.

Studies have shown that there was a 24 percent reduction in the rate of new STIs in groups of Thai sex workers who were given the choice of using either the male or female condom, compared with groups offered only the male condom. [5] There have been many studies of the use of the female condom in developing countries. Many have involved commercial sex workers who generally accept the device more quickly than other women. Most studies have shown high or moderate acceptability among sex workers, including those in China, Costa Rica,

C™te d'Ivoire, Thailand, and Zimbabwe.[6] But these studies also revealed a number of barriers to the use of the female condom, including clients' distrust of unfamiliar methods, inconvenience, insertion difficulties, discomfort or pain from the inner ring, and itching.

These obstacles can be overcome by the introduction of condoms, technical support and counseling. Women who have experience with the male condom or who receive more intensive training with the female condom generally find the device easier to use. Research in Zambia showed that the addition of female condoms with counseling on the barrier method mix could reduce unprotected sex among couples at high risk of HIV infection.[7] Marketing Strategies Social marketing has been used widely in the promotion of the male condom in developing countries and this strategy is now being applied to the female condom.

English for sex work

It is evident that if the client and the sex worker do not speak the same language, they will have problems in negotiating safe sex, more so when they are both intoxicated. The most logical intervention would therefore be to teach English to sex workers and the other actors involved in sex tourism. It is just as important to teach Spanish to customers. The most professional mongers are already in the process of learning the new language, but it is less likely that the causal sex tourist will master Spanish in a few days.

María wants to take conversational classes that relate to her work. "I want to learn how to ask for a "chupadita" (cunnilingus) in English. I don't need to learn that "María bakes a cake at home," she says with humor. She also indicated that with a better command of English, there would be fewer frictions with customers and a lesser risk of unsafe sex.

Miss Safe: interactive software

One complaint from sex tourists is the multiple problems they face in the bedroom: not knowing the sex worker's language, having difficulties with sex negotiation, shyness about discussing sexual practices and prices, cultural misunderstandings and alcohol intoxication.

To prevent any misunderstanding between the client and the sex worker an innovative approach was suggested in our discussions with mongers: to create a virtual character called Ms. Safe. This software could be installed in the hotel televisions. Once the client enters the room, the television will turn on and Ms. Safe will appear on the screen. She will serve as an English and Spanish translator. The purpose is to help the sex worker and the client with their sexual negotiations, especially when the two of them have consumed alcohol. The program –according to our interviewees– should include the following subjects:

- Price and duration of the encounter.
- Safe sexual practice preferred. Miss safe will not recommend any unprotected sexual practice.
- Erotic language preferred.
- Dress.
- Dance.
- Liquor consumption. Miss Safe will warn both users to limit alcohol consumption.
- Respect for sex worker.

The first step should be to create Miss Safe, an interactive character that would work as a mediator between the client and the customer. Miss Safe would translate phrases, provide alternatives, remind loggers of safe sex practices and would help overcome obstacles. Some sort of artificial intelligence should be introduced to allow more fluid conversations. She should express emotions through face gestures and should have a voice generator that allows fluidity in both Spanish and English. To complement verbal communication, texts and images should be added. Clients would be able to ask for information by selecting images in a touch–screen or in a game–pad. Both clients and sex workers would be able to agree on prices, sexual games and practices. Nevertheless, recommendations would follow on how to have them safely.

The program would include a complete user's registry to allow the generation of statistics on interaction, sexual preferences, communication problems and obstacles to safe sex. When Miss Safe is not able to answer a specific question, the program would direct the user to a human operator that would solve the problem.

A sex worker's website, paper and Guardian Angel program

In our discussions with sex workers, they suggested an interesting alternative to do harm reduction, empowerment and safe sex promotion. They proposed the creation of a Website and the publication of a magazine for sex workers and their clients. Mongers also were keen to the proposal, as they would like to have information on places to go, prices to pay, new sex alternatives and more importantly, a vehicle to learn and communicate with sex workers.

The website will help tourists, before coming to Costa Rica, on everything there is to know about Costa Rica's nightlife. It will allow them to chat with sex workers and to plan their future trip. It will also teach them about the problems that can arise with intoxication and drug consumption so that they can think of alternatives to prevent risks.

Nocturna: the sex worker's magazine

During the first RAP we asked about the acceptability of a newspaper or magazine geared to Costa Rica's nightlife. Sex workers thought they needed a vehicle to voice their concerns, to organize themselves, to get information on sex work and its risks, and to share their views with customers. They wanted the magazine to include also the customer's perspectives, their desires, their expectations and any information they wanted to share with the sex workers.

Mongers also found the idea attractive as they are always wondering what is going on in the women's minds. In several sex forums there were suggestions to create channels to communicate with sex workers. Both sex workers and mongers have provided with a possible name for the magazine: "*Nocturna*."

Guardian Angel program

Both sex workers and mongers proposed to start a program that would emulate a designated driver's program that helps people avoid driving under the influence. Women reasoned that they do not remember much when inebriated The same happens with men who admitted having serious problems in using condoms when drunk. The program will consist of paying some women and men to do the following tasks:

- Provide condoms in the premises.
- Assure that sex workers or customers do not get intoxicated.
- Speak with clients on the need to have safe sex and to respect sex workers prior their eloping to the rooms.
- Serve as a translator o mediator in case of problems.

Non–mandatory HIV testing

Mongers want sex workers to be tested but the women are hesitant about its benefits. Sex workers consider it only in case of pregnancy and to protect their children.

As a compromise, both groups agreed in having optional and confidential HIV testing. The test should be anonymous –according to the views expressed by sex workers in our discussions– and to be done at private labs, not associated with the Ministry of Health. [8] This would provide them with protection from police harassment and in the case of foreign workers, deportation. Mongers also do not want public officials doing the tests and would consider taking them only in private labs.

HIV testing can have benefits for the person who takes a test, their sexual partners and the wider community, provided that it is part of a package of prevention, counseling, care and support. It can lead to improved health and medical treatment, more informed decision–making, better practical and emotional support, increased motivation to prevent HIV transmission, and more positive attitudes towards living with HIV. It also would provide a clearance to work in the sex industry that infected sex workers would not receive. This will provide a good incentive to limit alcohol intoxication and unsafe sex.

People who know that they have HIV can take steps to protect themselves and sexual partners who may be uninfected. People who test negative can be counseled about how to avoid HIV infection. There is some evidence that HIV counseling and testing programs can motivate people to change to safer sexual behavior, if testing is voluntary and accompanied by high–quality post–test counseling, provision of condoms and ongoing care and support. [9]

Never has there been a preventive intervention or program for sex workers in the Costa Rica's sexual tourism industry. Moreover, the only ones that get tested are the ones working in brothels that cater to low–income men. As the tourist sex industry remains practically illegal, it is hard to expect a prevention program –as the one recommended above– to be implemented by the Costa Rican government.

Lupita, for example, thinks "The Costa Rican government would rather see us dead than admitting it has a huge prostitution problem." She knows that the State is so sex–negative and so much under the control of the Catholic hierarchy that it will not be able to talk to the women in a respectful manner. "The Government was not able to print the sex education school guides for adolescents given the Church's opposition. How are they going to do something for prostitutes?" –She asks.

Jack52 also believes that Costa Ricans would rather put mongers in prison than to talk to them.

> *The Catholic Church will never allow any prevention program either among upper class prostitutes or sex tourists. When sex workers came to Costa Rica*

from all over the world for a Congress on HIV prevention some years ago, the Church sent its troops made of fundamental Christians to prevent the event from taking place. When a Lesbian meeting was to be held in San José, the Interior Minister sent the police to "spot" lesbians at the airport and prevent them from entering the country. Any woman who traveled alone was a suspect. Perhaps with mongers, they will do something similar. Any American man who is old, fat and heads to San José instead of the beach, will be stopped, his bags searched for condoms and women's perfumes, and if he has a picture of a girl who is dark looking and her name is Carmen, be deported to the States. [10]

Nevertheless, as more middle–class seniors in the United States become infected with the HIV virus, perhaps the motivation will come from the places that helped to develop this third world country's sex tourist economy.

Notes

1. Johnny Madrigal and Jacobo Schifter, *Encuesta Nacional de Sida,* San José: Asociación Demográfica Costarricense, 1990.
2. Ibid.
3. Johnny Madrigal, Jacobo Schifter, and Paul Feldblum, "Female Condom Acceptability Among Sex Workers in Costa Rica," AIDS Education and Prevention 10, no. 2 (1998): 105–13
4. World Health Organization (WHO), *Women and HIV/AIDS,* fact sheet no. 242 (Geneva: WHO, 2002)
5. A.L. Fontanet et al., "Protection Against Sexually Transmitted Diseases by Granting Sex Workers in Thailand the Choice of Using the Male or Female Condom: Results from a Randomized Controlled Trial," AIDS 12, no. 14 (1998)
6. A.L. Fontanet et al., "Protection Against Sexually Transmitted Diseases by Granting Sex Workers in Thailand the Choice of Using the Male or Female Condom: Results from a Randomized Controlled Trial," AIDS 12, no. 14 (1998): 1851–59. 16. Francois Deniaud, "ActualitÎ du prÎservatif fÎminin en Afrique," SantÎ 7, no. 6 (1997): 405–15. 17. C. Yimin et al., "Introductory Study on Female Condom Use Among Sex Workers in China," Contraception 66, no. 3 (2002): 179–85. Johnny Madrigal, Jacobo Schifter, and Paul Feldblum, "Female Condom Acceptability Among Sex Workers in Costa Rica," AIDS Education and Prevention 10, no. 2 (1998): 105–13. Francois Deniaud, "Dynamiques d'acceptabilitÎ du prÎservatif fÎminin chez des prostituÎes et des jeunes femmes ˆ Abidjan, C™te d'Ivoire," Migrations SantÎ 94–95 (1997): 111–37. 20.Sunanda Ray et al., "Constraints Faced by Sex Workers in Use of Female and Male Condoms for Safer Sex in Urban Zimbabwe," Journal of Urban Health 78, no. 4 (2001): 581–92. United Nations Population Fund (UNFPA), "Condom Programming for HIV Prevention," HIV Prevention Now, Programme Briefs (New York: UNFPA, 2002).
7. Sohail Agha, "Intention to Use the Female Condom Following a Mass–Marketing, Zambia," American Journal of Public Health 91, no. 2 (2001): 307–10.

8. Policy Paper on the Forced Testing and Quarantining of Prostitutes. Prostitutes Safe Sex Project (Maggies). Toronto: The Project, 1993; English Collective of Prostitutes. Prostitute Women and AIDS: Resisting the Virus of Repression. San Francisco, CA: PROstitutes Collective, 1988 (US edition). See also Sex Industry and the AIDS Debate '88. Report and Conference Papers from the First National Sex Industry Conference, Melbourne, Australia, 25–27 October 1988. St Kilda, Victoria: Prostitutes Collective of Victoria, 1988.

9. In Uganda, the AIDS Information and Counselling Centre found that clients reported increases in condom use from 10 percent to 89 per cent with regular partners and from 28 per cent to 100 per cent with casual partners. A recent study in Tanzania, Kenya and Trinidad found that rates of condom use or number of sexual partners were associated with knowledge of HIV–positive status, high quality counselling and provision of condoms. http://www.aidsaction.info/ht/section1.html

10. http://www.costaricaticas.com/phpbb2/viewtopic.php?t=3500

Epilogue

North Americans who participate in sexual tourism do not travel, unlike Christopher Columbus, to invent, impose or create something new in the tropics. Our aborigines are not those genuine and naïve beings on the tricks and stratagems of occidental culture that can be easily bought with small shampoo bottles from visited hotel rooms. Neither are gringos, monsters of world imperialism that destroy local cultures and the good customs of the new markets that they invade. We could say that they make use of what is already there and look for relationships that ticos and ticas have already established among themselves. Prostitution in our country has colonial origins therefore it existed before American sex tourists began to take notice of it. Contrary to popular belief, they also did not thrust the obsession for sex and the absence of clear life goals. American sex tourists found in Costa Rican a society without course and without alternatives for something to do rather than seducing each other and abandoning ourselves in search for the ultimate orgasm. A culture that is inundated with lies, simulation, consumption, credit, hyperreality and the wretched relations between men and women. "Monguers" only benefit from what is already available in our medium.

"Thank you for being with us and letting us into your homes" –Pilar Cisnero, a television broadcaster from one of the main news channel in the country tells us while she directly looks into the camera and gives us a cordial smile. However, Pilar is not really looking at us nor was she invited into our homes. We have only turned on the television and probably did not have another choice but to watch her. Pilar, in turn, directs herself to a cold machine with lots of make–up to project a natural look since television distorts the skins normal pigment. Minutes after this same program, a Mastercard commercial tells us that in life there are things that money cannot buy, but for everything else there is the credit card. However, what we can not buy, according to the commercial, are the special moments that our loved ones give us when we give what we can buy them. Would the grandmother from the commercial still love us if we did not bring her the strawberries? Further on, the president of the republic communicates of the government's program and that his biggest preoccupation is the poor and the country, when we all know that this is not true, that no candidate cares about a sea of indigents with whom they would never socialize with. In the health's news section, a journalist covers a report about married women who get breast implants. Housewives that have lived for 5, 10 or 20 years with their partners decide to go through the operation to feel themselves and their partners in "love" again. Nobody explains how someone can become erotic all of a sudden with breast that have never been there for 5, 10 or 20 years. In a report on articles for the home, a plant with leaves made out of silk look so real that the housekeeper waters it believing it is real. Later on, the newscast informs on how in a dentist clinic, we can get our teeth whitened with acids to make them look as if they were new. Finally, after the news, a soap opera convinces us that Maria desperately loves Carlos and that he in turn cares for her even though he acts like he does not since he was told that Maria did not love him and with his indifference he punishes her. Maria, in turn, did love him but when she is treated with indifference she also acts like she does not care about him.

What are we talking about? According to Baudrilliard, it is about simulation and it has arrived to the tropics. Simulation makes fantasies seem real to the degree that we do not know what is or is not real. Pilar's greeting, the Mastercard commercial, the President's briefing, silicon breasts, the artificial Taiwanese plants, whitened teeth and the love of the actors in the soap opera, although fake, seem real without mattering if they are or not. The same happens with sex worker's orgasms, GFE relationships, the tears at the airport, the second houses, the fishing trips and the weddings at Hotel Mamei. Everything is a simulation, making something appear that it is. Today's prostitution is simply one more representation of a theatrical sometimes romantic play that makes us belief in love when there is none. And what about if there is? Who cares? And if there is not, as Astroglide questioned, who loses their sleep?

The sexual tourism boom is simply simulation that not only involves the principal actors but also those that benefit from it. Simulation historically arrived with the advent of capitalism. The reason for this is because this economic system makes us belief that happiness can be bought. It lies in the newest car in the market or the purchase of a gorgeous house that will probably take you 20 years to pay due to the draining credits from a bank that calls itself our friend. And although none of this makes us happy, we simulate that it does since it took us so much hard work to acquire. A culture that lives on simulation is one that has lost its truths and its realities. Our culture is so false that we do not even realize it. If you do not believe me, ask the monkeys at Manual Antonio's

National Park that only eat from what the tourists give them and simulate to be wild animals only to benefit from the park's visitors. Recently, three thousand monkeys died of unknown causes; they probably took a bottle of Viagra that was left forgotten.

In a televised soccer game between Saprissa and La Liga, an announcer states what is happening even though we are all watching the game with our own eyes. Nevertheless, the announcer is crucial to the game and cannot be omitted; we are all waiting for his cries when there is a goal. Furthermore, the television gives us the opportunity to watch the game from different (camera) angles, perspectives that a spectator in the stadium misses. So why go to the stadium to watch a game if we can see it better on television? In the other hand, an adolescent buys an ipod and can listen to a rock concert so well and with the capacity to vary its decibels in such a manner that not even in the concert could he appreciate its quality of sound. Maria tattooed her eyebrows so they can always look dashing, something regular makeup cannot emulate. Jose and Carla got married. They were so nervous in their wedding that wanted it to be over so they could enjoy it in their video.

What is this an example of? According to Baudrilliard, it is hyper reality or to make reality more intense and dramatic to a degree that it feels better than life itself. The goals praised by the soccer announcer, the music in the ipod, the tattoo and videos that provide us with a reality that is more beautiful, more detailed that what our senses can provide us. In a beautiful picture or in a detailed movie, sweat, bad odors, gases, tensions, anxiety are all missing. All these and other annoyances of our biological reality that remind us that happiness does not last more than an evening in spring. The same happens with sex and the tricks to make it hyperreal: the bed stunts, orgies, theatrical works, filming, drugs, screams and the hotels like El Mamei.

Prostitution is sex better than sex since it is free of emotions and feelings that make all human relations something imperfect and finite. In sexual tourism, there is no disillusion because there is no jealousy, the fear of abandonment, the unexpected treason, and the most important, boredom. "Monguers" come accompanied by cameras and videos, dildos and paraphernalia that allow the sexual act to be seen and experienced in a way impossible with just our sexual organs. Sex tourists take Viagra, Cialis or Levitra and can have sexual relations that last more than the Energizer bunny.

Why do we want so much hyperreality? A simple answer would be so gringos, ticos and ticas can lessen the degree of boredom and if we still are bored of life is because there is no good reason for not being. What used to console us like paradise and a loving God that was looking after us with open arms, does not anymore. Neither does the acquisition of material things since they end indebting and economically ruining us.

So what is left? Sex. Its actual dominion cannot be placed on North Americans since Costa Rican society, after so many years of Puritanism and a double moral, has begun to look in this salvation. Political, religious and ideological disillusionment have left us with nothing. A priest murdered a journalist that accused him of profiting at the expense of the people; two ex–presidents ended in jail for corruption; a feminist congressman orders, with government money, to make a paved road that only leads to her home; union syndicalists who call themselves leaders of the poor party a Monday night with money from the people. We are so fed up with all this that we do not even notice it anymore.

We now only live for sex. We define ourselves by objects or the practice of desired sex. We talk unstoppably about the subject in the most conservative places. Furthermore we believe that in sex there lie the new Messiahs that will take us out of underdevelopment, stagnation and the boring life of working to simply pay the bills. Sex is overvalued. It now has a historic responsibility and has substituted the mystic experiences of long ago; we live in search of the last orgasm before leaving this unjust world. After all this, is the only thing that is left that provides us with some pleasure and that it does not disillusion or betrays like everything else.

Obviously, globalization ties us with an international economy that promotes the specialization of each country. In Latin countries, we have concentrated more and more in our genital organs. If in agriculture and manufacturing our hands and feet gave us something to eat; now it is our penises and our vaginas. In the case of Costa Rica, whether we like it or not, sexual tourism is an important component of our GDP. We are a country that is cheaper and populated by what is considered to be "the other" and the "natural" for white Americans and Europeans. Now, we are converting in their sexual servants and this does not only include sex workers, but all other from the person that receives them in the airport to the one that sends them off. Although this is not the topic of this book, it is no secret that nongovernmental organizations, like what happened with Casa Alianza, and private banks promote sexuality as a form of payment and contributions to the third world. (Some day I would like to write about the experiences of European and American donors of developing countries and how the latter expect "sexual favors" from the former as a sign of their generosity). Or how it usually happens in private companies where responsibilities demand more than personal assistance. Or in the same universities where female students tend to unbutton their shirts before male professors to pass a course or male students that after failing a class accept a personal invitation from their female professor to see what they can do about it. Prostitution and its different forms of it, threatened to disintegrate relations since it is impossible to have mutual respect for one another when one is obliged to perform oral sex.

Prostitution is greatly tied to the changes of sexual roles. Female liberation has struggled to find equality through the law and in doing so has estimated female contributions to the home in monetary terms lessening the frontier between heterosexual marriage and prostituted relations. In both cases, sexuality has a price, be it with money or food pensions. The ever increasing role of the state, from the United States and also Costa Rica, to punish unfaithful husbands and those that do not pay child support has led more American and Costa Rican men to look for prostitutes. This has indirectly led to prostitution since men now look for uncompromising relationships. "Monguers" complain that their partners take advantage of them and live at their expense. They look for sex workers since they do not want assertive or "liberated" women. Prostituted relationships are "traditional" in the sense that men and women act as opposites. It is a struggle against the tendency to make us more alike than different. Ironically, in sexual tourism, "machista" and "traditional" men play the roles of romantic and sensitive gentleman and strong and decisive women act as if they were submissive and helpless. The most ironic thing is that in this profession women are able to become economically independent, manage their own money and live lives that some feminists would even envy. This proves that nothing is what it seems.

Finally, sexual tourism is a threat to the spread of HIV/AIDS unless there is a prevention program that is respectful of sex workers and their client's human rights. Intimacy not ignorance is the main culprit in the spread of the virus. If sexual tourism would only be about sex, and would not have the love component, then there would be fewer dangers to contracting HIV. What starts as a simple commercial relationship is complicated and can turn to something real than can lead to death. To implement an effective prevention program, it is important to create a fictional character –Ms Segura – that simulates to care for the health of both men and women. This virtual woman will have the mission to save lives that human beings of flesh and bones, in view of the stigmatization of prostitution, would not care to rescue.

Annex, charts, graphics and diagrams

Table 1 **Major sources of generating revenues in Costa Rica, (in U.S. million of dollars) from 1990 to 2002**

Year	Tourism	Coffee	Banana	Meat	Sugar
1990	275,0	245,4	315,0	48,6	25,1
1991	330,6	263,6	396,6	69,3	24,7
1992	431,1	201,6	562,6	44,0	29,5
1993	577,4	201,6	564,8	63,7	27,9
1994	625,7	307,6	561,0	51,0	28,6
1995	659,6	417,1	680,2	43,6	46,1
1996	688,6	385,4	631,1	42,2	44,4
1997	719,3	402,3	577,3	28,3	41,1
1998	883,5	409,5	667,5	24,0	41,8
1999	1036,1	288,7	629,0	27,2	30,0
2000	1229,2	273,7	546,1	30,7	28,6
2001	1095,5	161,8	515,9	25,5	35,5
2002	1078,0	165,1	478,4	20,1	27,0

Source: CANATUR, Dirección de Investigación, based on Tourist Board's data.
http://www.canatur.org/80fb514e3dce55c3edc2edf998345425/estadisticas/33
Consultation Date: 08-23-04

Table 2 **Motivations for travel to Costa Rica (percentage distribution of interviewed passengers regardless of nationality) from 1997 to 2002**

Motive	1997	1998	1999	2000	2001	2002
Relative Total	100,0	100,0	100,0	100,0	100,0	100,0
Vacation, recreation, pleasure	73,7	64,8	65,4	61,5	68,0	61,3
Visits to family and/or friends	3,8	6,7	4,5	8,4	11,5	23,7
Business or work	13,7	18,3	22,7	21,7	13,5	10,0
Study	4,0	3,8	3,3	3,8	1,8	3,0
Other motives	4,8	6,4	4,1	4,6	5,2	2,0

Source: CANATUR, Dirección de Investigación, based on Tourist Board's data.
http://www.canatur.org/80fb514e3dce55c3edc2edf998345425/estadisticas/41
Consultation Date: 08-23-04

Table 3 **Number of tourists from the US and method of travel from 1990 to 2002**

Year	By Air	By Land	By Sea	Total
1990	144329	4857	1038	150224
1991	165493	6440	1693	173626
1992	208069	7924	1700	217693
1993	231745	8538	2263	242546
1994	251969	9491	2108	263568
1995	272151	11458	3825	287434
1996	255439	12244	3618	271301
1997	268906	12050	4405	285361
1998	329042	13125	5275	347442
1999	368644	16585	7327	392556
2000	396909	14101	18715	429725
2001	403775	16667	8651	429093
2002	400758	16914	4543	422215
Total	3697229	150394	65161	3912784

Source: CANATUR, Dirección de Investigación, based on Tourist Board's data.
http://www.canatur.org/80fb514e3dce55c3edc2edf998345425/estadisticas/1
http://www.canatur.org/80fb514e3dce55c3edc2edf998345425/estadisticas/2
http://www.canatur.org/80fb514e3dce55c3edc2edf998345425/estadisticas/3
http://www.canatur.org/80fb514e3dce55c3edc2edf998345425/estadisticas/4
Consultation Date: 08-23-04

Table 4 **Costa Rica: Commercial sex workers, sociodemographic variables**

Characteristics		1997 Study	2000 Study
	(N)	(300)	(400)
	Total	100.0	100.0
Age			
Less than 20		12.3	7.3
20 - 24		21.3	24.0
25 - 29		2.3	22.0
30 - 34		16.7	16.5
35 - 39		13.7	13.5
40 and more		15.7	17.0
Education			
Unfinished primary or less		32.1	23.5
Completed primary		24.1	26.3
Unfinished high school		36.1	39.3
High school completed		5.4	7.5
University studies		2.3	3.5
% knows how to read		92.0	92.0
% knows how to write		88.7	91.5
Civil status			
Single		54.0	57.3
Cohabiting		26.0	21.8
Married		2.3	3.8
Others		17.7	17.1
Number of children			
0		11.4	6.8
1		22.1	25.5
2		24.1	26.0
3		20.1	6.8
4		9.0	12.8
5 - 6		9.7	8.8
7 and more		3.7	3.5

Average [1]	2.5	2.5
Mode	2.0	2.0
Median	2.0	2.0
Degree of religion devotion		
None	17.3	14.5
Little	37.7	30.0
Regular	23.0	28.8
Lots	22.0	26.3
Religion		
Catholic	66.0	65.1
Evangelical	23.3	21.7
None	6.3	10.7
Others	4.7	2.5

1. All resume measurements were calculated using gross values of variables.

Table 5 **Costa Rica: Commercial sex workers, socioeconomic indicators**

Indicators		1997 Study	200 Study
	(N)	(300)	(400)
	Total	100.0	100.0
Monthly income in dollars			
Less than 200		32.3	25.8
200 to less than 400		37.3	37.5
400 to less than 600		16.7	19.0
600 to less than 800		7.3	10.8
800 to less than 1000		5.0	4.3
1000 to less than 1500		1.0	1.0
1500 and more		0.3	1.8
Average [1]		331.1	384.1
Mode		332.0	323.0
Median		249.0	323.0
Ownership of appliances [2]			
Color TV		71.0	84.5
Refrigerator		65.3	71.8
Washing machine		69.7	68.5
Microwave		16.7	22.0
VHS		25.0	33.3
Cellular phone		---	10.5
Computer		---	4.5
Car (not for work)		5.0	6.0
Socioeconomic index [3]			
(without cellular phone and computer)			
Average		10.7	6.0
Mode		9.9	4.1
Median		9.6	4.1
Socioeconomic index [4]			
(with cellular phone and computer)			
Average		---	8.0
Mode		---	4.1
Median		---	4.1

Number of dependents		
0	14.0	4.3
1	16.0	13.8
2	19.3	16.8
3	13.7	24.8
4	14.7	16.5
5 - 6	14.3	16.5
7 - 8	6.3	4.8
10 and more	1.7	2.8
Average [1]	3.0	3.4
Mode	2.0	3.0
Median	3.0	3.0

Average price for clients		
Less than 10	---	67.5
10 - 19	---	30.5
20 - 29	---	0.5
30 - 49	---	1.0
50 - 99	---	0.0
100 and more	---	0.5
Average [1]	---	9.1
Mode	---	6.0
Median	---	7.0

Have you been trained for a job?		
Yes	42.5	41.8
No	57.5	58.2

1 All resume measurements were calculated using gross values of variables.

2 Not referred to percent distribution, but to the percent that answered affirmatively of the totality of interviewed.

3 To calculate (I) index it was applied the formula I = xi Pi-1, where xi is a dichotomy variable meaning the ownership or not of appliance "i" and Pi is the percentage of ownership of each appliance. For the year 1997, the minimum value of index is 0.0 and the maximum is 37. At 2000, the respective values are 0.0 and 28.3

4 The minimum value of index is 0.0 and the maximum is 60.0

Table 6 Costa Rica: Commercial sex workers, place of birth and residence

Characteristics		1997 Study	2000 Study
	(N)	(300)	(400)
	Total	100.0	100.0
Was born in...			
Metropolitan area		42.7	37.8
Outside metropolitan area		56.7	62.3
Don't know		0.7	0.0
Actually lives in...			
Metropolitan area		84.7	83.2
Outside metropolitan area		15.3	16.8
Number of years living in area			
Less than 5		47.7	31.8
5 - 9		19.7	17.8
10 - 19		18.7	21.3
20 - 29		9.3	15.5
30 - 39		3.0	8.8
40 - 49		1.0	4.5
50 and more		0.7	0.5
Average1		9.1	13.4
Mode		0.0	0.0
Median		6.0	10.0

1 All resume measurements were calculated using gross values of variables.

Table 7 **Costa Rica: Commercial sex workers, work related aspects**

Aspects		1997 Study	200 Study
	(N)	(300)	(400)
	Total	100.0	100.0
How do you label your work?			
Woman in prostitution		3.7	2.8
Prostitute		24.3	20.0
Sex worker		31.0	42.8
Sexual worker		5.7	11.8
Woman of "ambiente"		17.0	---
"Meretriz"		0.7	0.0
Other		16.0	16.3
Does not respond		1.7	6.5
Number of years in this job			
Less than 1		15.0	0.0
1 - 2		24.7	39.3
3 - 4		16.0	16.0
5 - 6		9.3	10.5
7 - 8		7.7	6.8
9 and more		27.7	27.3
Average [1]		3.3	1.9
Mode		0.0	1.0
Median		1.0	1.0
Current sexual practice			
Only men		93.7	90.5
Men and occasionally women		3.0	5.3
Men and women		3.3	4.0
Women and occasionally men		0.0	0.3
Only women		0.0	0.0

1 All resume measurements were calculated using gross values of variables.

Table 8 **Costa Rica: Commercial sex workers, drug consumption**

Variables		1997 Study	2000 Study
	(N)	(300)	(400)
	Total	100.0	100.0
% that drinks alcohol		63.0	57.8
Patterns of consumption			
Every day		15.0	10.3
More than twice a week		4.7	5.8
One or twice a week		19.0	15.5
One or twice a month		9.0	8.3
Seldom		15.3	18.0
Never		31.0	31.0
Abstinence		6.0	11.3
% of those who have consumed drugs		51.7	38.0
Marihuana		36.7	26.0
Cocaine		33.7	26.0
Smoked cocaine		18.0	10.0
Inhaled cocaine		31.0	24.0
Injected cocaine		3.7	1.0
Cement		11.7	3.8
Crack		20.3	10.5
Amphetamines		11.0	2.5
Hallucinogenic mushrooms		7.0	2.0
Heroine		2.0	0.0
Smoked heroine		1.7	0.0
Injected heroine		1.7	0.0
Other		11.3	0.0
% of those who currently consume drugs		27.7	13.0
Marihuana		10.3	18.3
Cocaine		8.7	8.0
Smoked cocaine		4.7	25.0
Inhaled cocaine		8.7	21.8
Injected cocaine		0.7	25.0
Cement		9.0	31.0

Crack	1.0	0.0
Amphetamines	2.0	20.0
Hallucinogenic mushrooms	0.3	0.0
Heroine	0.3	0.0
Smoked heroine	0.0	0.0
Injected heroine	0.7	0.0
Other	9.7	0.0

Patterns of current drug consumption		
Every day	---	54.0
More than twice a week	---	10.0
One or twice a week	---	16.0
One or twice a month	---	8.0
Not every frequently	---	12.0

Table 9 Costa Rica: Commercial sex workers, drug consumption and sexual practice

Variables	1997 Study	2000 Study
(N)	(300)	(400)
% who combines occasionally alcohol and sex	32.3	48.9
% who has problems using condoms when drinking	11.0	71.2
% who combines drugs and sex	15.0	10.0
% who has problems using condoms when taking drugs	---	13.5

Table 10 **Costa Rica: Commercial sex workers, percentage who did not use condom with men during last 12 months**

Sexual practice		1997 Study	2000 Study
	(N)	(300)	(400)
1. Has been penetrated by the vagina without condom		71.0	40.3
2. Has been penetrated by the anus without condom		12.0	9.3
3. Has ejaculated in mouth without condom		13.7	14.0
Non - use condom index (1+2)		71.0	40.8
Non - use condom index (1+2+3)		71.7	42.8

Note: To calculate the index of non use condoms, it was verified for each interviewed at least one of the mentioned practices occurred.

Table 11 **Costa Rica: Commercial sex workers, sex with regular clients**

Regular clients		1997 Study	2000 Study
	(N)	(300)	(400)
	Total	100.0	100.0
Number of regular clients during last month			
0		5.3	8.3
1-19		93.7	66.8
20-49		0.3	23.5
50-99		0.3	1.3
100-199		0.0	0.0
200 and more		0.0	0.3
Average [1]		1.0	11.8
Mode		0.8	10.0
Median		0.4	10.0
Number of clients who do not want to use condoms			
0		---	31.1
1-4		---	40.3
5-9		---	18.8
10-19		---	7.4
20 and more		---	2.5
Average [1]		---	3.7
Mode		---	0.0
Median		---	2.0
	(N)	(281)	(367)
	Total	100.0	100.0
Did the last regular client use condom last time you had sex?			
Yes		80.9	94.0
No		19.9	6.0

1 All resume measurements were calculated using gross values of variables.

Table 12 Costa Rica: Commercial sex workers, sex with occasional clients

Occasional clients		1997 Study	2000 Study
	(N)	(300)	(400)
	Total	100.0	100.0
Number of occasional clients during last month			
Less than 10		15.0	15.5
10 - 19		7.9	13.5
20 - 29		9.7	24.1
30 - 39		9.4	12.5
40 - 49		7.3	11.3
50 - 99		24.1	15.5
100 and more		25.0	7.8
Average [1]		78.1	36.5
Mode		86.7	20.0
Median		49.5	25.0
Number of occasional clients who do not want to use condoms			
0		---	10.0
1-4		---	34.2
5-9		---	34.4
10-19		---	13.6
20 - 49		---	5.9
50 and more		---	1.8
Average [1]		---	6.8
Mode		---	5.0
Median		---	5.0
	(N)	(296)	(382)
	Total	100.0	100.0
Did the last occasional client use condom last time you had sex?			
Yes		89.5	95.5
No		10.5	4.5

1 All resume measurements were calculated using gross values of variables.

Table 13 **Costa Rica: Commercial sex workers, what they do when regular clients refuse to use condoms**

Aspects		1997 Study	2000 Study
	(N)	(300)	(400)
	Total	100.0	100.0
Reject him			
Yes, spontaneous		---	74.9
Yes, with support		---	8.4
No		---	16.6
Not to practice penetration			
Yes, spontaneous		---	2.7
Yes, with support		---	12.0
No		---	85.3
Put condom without client's knowledge			
Yes, spontaneous		---	1.4
Yes, with support		---	8.7
No		---	89.9
Charges him more			
Yes, spontaneous		---	0.5
Yes, with support		---	10.6
No		---	88.8
Gives client to other sex worker			
Yes, spontaneous		---	0.5
Yes, with support		---	17.7
No		---	81.7
Gives in to client			
Yes, spontaneous		---	4.4
Yes, with support		---	11.7
No		---	83.9

Table 14 **Costa Rica: Commercial sex workers, what they do when occasional clients refuse to use condoms**

Aspects		1997 Study	2000 Study
	(N)	(300)	(400)
	Total	100.0	100.0
Reject him			
Yes, spontaneous		---	81.0
Yes, with support		---	6.2
No		---	12.9
Not to practice penetration			
Yes, spontaneous		---	1.5
Yes, with support		---	12.6
No		---	85.9
Put condom without client's knowledge			
Yes, spontaneous		---	0.3
Yes, with support		---	8.7
No		---	91.0
Charges him more			
Yes, spontaneous		---	1.0
Yes, with support		---	9.5
No		---	89.5
Gives client to other sex worker			
Yes, spontaneous		---	1.5
Yes, with support		---	17.5
No		---	81.0
Gives in to client			
Yes, spontaneous		---	2.8
Yes, with support		---	11.6
No		---	85.6

Table 15 Costa Rica: Commercial sex workers, sex and condom use in intimate relationships

Aspects		1997 Study	200 Study
	(N)	(300)	(400)
	Total	100.0	100.0
% of those who had intimate relationships [1]		66.7	56.8
% cohabitating [2]		50.3	47.3
% in other intimate relationships [3]		27.0	18.0
	(N)	(200)	(227)
All who shared intimate relationships without being paid			
% who did not use condom		79.0	48.0
	(N)	(151)	(189)
Cohabitating			
% who did not use condom		76.2	41.0
	(N)	(200)	(227)
Others			
% who did not use condom		72.8	12.5

1 Referred to a sexual relation with people than clients, such as husband, partner, boyfriend or fried.
2 Married or cohabitating.
3 Boyfriend, friend.

Table 16 Costa Rica: Commercial sex workers, condom use with regular clients

Condom use		1997 Study	200 Study
	(N)	(300)	(400)
	Total	100.0	100.0
% of those who ever used condoms		98.3	99.8
	(N)	(295)	(399)
	Total	100.0	100.0
Do you use condoms currently?			
Yes		99.0	99.5
No		1.0	0.5
How frequent?			
Always		66.1	86.4
Almost always		21.7	8.6
Sometimes		9.5	4.8
Almost never		2.7	0.3
Who decides to use it?			
She		86.1	89.9
Client		5.8	3.5
Both		3.4	4.0
Sometimes him, sometimes her		4.7	2.5
Do you use condom to prevent STI´s?			
Yes, spontaneous		93.5	92.4
Yes, with support		5.8	6.5
No		0.7	1.0
Do you use condom to prevent AIDS?			
Yes, spontaneous		71.2	82.9
Yes, with support		26.4	16.1
No		2.4	1.0

Do you use condom for hygienic reason?		
Yes, spontaneous	17.3	20.5
Yes, with support	78.0	74.2
No	4.7	5.3

Do you use condom to prevent pregnancies?		
Yes, spontaneous	38.1	25.7
Yes, with support	23.1	26.2
No	38.8	48.1

Table 17 Costa Rica: Commercial sex workers, condom use with current partner

Condom use		1997 Study	200 Study
	(N)	(300)	(400)
	Total	100.0	100.0
% who has a partner		42.4	28.5
	(N)	(125)	(114)
	Total	100.0	100.0
Do you use condoms currently?			
Yes		17.6	14.2
No		82.4	85.8
How frequent?			
Always		9.6	7.6
Almost always		3.2	2.7
Sometimes		3.2	1.8
Almost never		1.6	1.8
Do not use it		82.4	85.8
Who decides to use it?			
She		63.6	56.3
Partner		---	6.3
Both		36.4	37.5
Do you use condom to prevent STI´s?			
Yes, spontaneous		11.2	10.7
Yes, with support		3.2	3.6
No		3.2	0.0
Do not use it		82.4	85.8
Do you use condom to prevent AIDS?			
Yes, spontaneous		9.6	7.6
Yes, with support		4.8	5.3
No		3.2	0.9
Do not use it		82.4	85.8

Do you use condom for hygienic reason?			
Yes, spontaneous		4.8	3.6
Yes, with support		10.4	8.0
No		20.4	25.7
Do not use it		82.4	85.8
Do you use condom to prevent pregnancies?			
Yes, spontaneous		7.2	8.0
Yes, with support		4.8	1.8
No		5.6	4.4
Do not use it		82.4	85.8

Table 18 Costa Rica: Commercial sex workers, obstacles to safe sex

Obstacles		1997 Study	2000 Study
	(N)	(300)	(400)
	Total	100	100
Do you feel or would you feel embarrassed to by condoms?			
Feel or would feel shame		18.3	17.5
Sometimes		2.7	1.6
Does not feel shame		77.6	70.5
Does not buy them		1.4	10.5
Do condoms decrease sexual pleasure?			
Yes, it does		41.0	39.8
Sometimes yes, sometimes not		44.0	3.3
Does not decrease it		2.3	47.0
Does not matter, only uses it		12.7	10.0
Broken condoms to partner or himself during last 12 months			
0		19.3	60.3
1		11.9	13.5
2		10.2	10.8
3 - 4		8.8	5.8
5 - 9		8.5	5.8
10 and more		1.2	4.0

Average general [1]	2.3	1.3
Summary of broken condoms		
Average	4.5	3.2
Mode	1.0	1.0
Median	3.0	2.0
Circumstances to drop condoms		
1. If alcohol is consumed	7.1	4.8
2. If person is known	22.7	16.0
3. If has sex with partner	66.4	60.7
4. If other does not ejaculate inside	18.1	12.3
5. If he penetrates without ejaculating inside	12.1	9.5
6. If practices oral sex	14.8	9.8
7. If practices masturbation	---	20.5

1 All resume measurements were calculated using gross values of variables.

Table 19 **Costa Rica: Commercial sex workers, correct condon use**

Correct use		1997 Study	200 Study
	(N)	(300)	(400)
% who participated in exercise		99.0	93.8
	(N)	(297)	(375)
Evaluated aspects			
1. Broke envelop with teeth		---	26.7
2. Broke envelop with sharp object		---	0.3
3. Broke envelop with finger on corner		69.7	60.2
4. Check expiration date		---	2.9
5. Check for air bubbles		---	24.8
6. Squeezed rip of condom extract air		57.6	28.0
7. Unrolled condom with fingers until base of dildo		93.2	71.0
8. Put lubricant on condom / rectum		70.4	28.7
9. With drew condom while holding ring		85.5	53.0
Correct use 1 (3+6+7)			
Correct use 2 (3+6+7+9)		49.2	18.5
Correct use 3 (3+6+7+8+9)		46.1	11.4
Correct use 4 (1a+2b+3)		31.3	4.0
Correct use 5 (1a+2b +3+4+7+9)		---	51.3
Correct use 6 (1a+2b +3+4+7+8+9)		---	2.0
Correct use 7 (1a+2b +3+4+5+6+7+8+9)		---	0.8

Note: To estimate the correct use of condom it was verified that each interviewed executes accurately the evaluated items.

a. Because this variable is evaluated in a positive way in the questionnaire, to include it in the index we use its complementary value.

b. Because this variable is evaluated in a positive way in the questionnaire, to include it in the index we use its complementary value.

Table 20 Costa Rica: Commercial sex workers, female condom

Aspects		1997 Study	200 Study
	(N)	(300)	(400)
Have you heard of female condom?		81.0	80.8
Have you ever used it?		27.0	44.1
Do you currently use it?		7.4	42.1

Table 21 Costa Rica: STI´s and HIV infections according to sex and region. First 26 weeks, 2004

	HIV infections			STI´s infections		
Region	Male	Female	Total	Male	Female	Total
Metropolitan Area	8	6	14	107	111	218
North Central	18	8	26	130	70	200
South Central	2	3	5	40	19	59
Chorotega Region	5	3	8	55	32	87
Huetar Atlántica Region	0	1	1	94	36	130
Huetar Northern Region	0	1	1	16	19	35
Total	33	22	55	442	287	729

Source: Programa de Análisis y Vigilancia Epiodemiológica. Caja Costarricense de Seguro Social. Date: September 2004.

Table 22 HIV prevalence in Central America

Country	Adult HIV prevalence %, end 2001	Men:Female Ratio AIDS cases 2001	HIV prevalence in female sex workers by place of work. 2001/02 (sample size)[1]	HIV prevalence in Men who have sex with men 2001/02 (sample size)[2]
Belize	2,0	0,8:1	N/A	N/A
Honduras	1,6	1,2:1	10,4	13,0
Panama	1,5	3:1	1,9	10,6
Guatemala	1,0	2,5:1	5,2	11,5
El Salvador	0,6	3:1	3,9	17,7
Costa Rica	0,6	7:1	N/A	N/A
Nicaragua	0,2	4:1	0,4	9,3

Source: HIV/AIDS in Central America: An Overview of Epidemic and Priorities for Prevention. Latin American and Caribbean Region. Global HIV/AIDS Program. World Bank, September 2003.

1 PASCA Multisite Study on STI´s and HIV probabilistic sample in capital cities census in port cities.

2 Sample is not representative, but rather drawn from men who volunteered to be tested, after seeingflyers and other promotion about the study from PASCA Multisite Study on STI´s and HIV.

Table 23 **STI´s absolute numbers of registered cases 1970, 1975, 1980, 1985, 1990 to 2003**

Year	Gonorrhea	Siphylis	Chancro blando	Urethritis no gonocócica	AIDS
1970*	2806	947	---	---	0
1975*	2813	1471	---	---	0
1980*	10898	2266	---	---	0
1985*	8286	1514	---	---	6
1990*	4274	1939	---	---	79
1991*	3683	1270	---	---	94
1992	3937	1781	135	2347	127
1993	1815	981	77	573	127
1994	2072	1184	122	946	171
1995	2305	1502	257	1086	208
1996	1911	1279	231	774	186
1997	1987	1452	145	556	177
1998	2124	1391	113	561	284
1999	1945	905	84	471	219
2000	1317	782	42	99	275
2001	1278	796	43	80	150
2002	1487	760	55	109	84
2003*	119	761	---	---	113

Source: Proyecto Estado de la Nación en Desarrollo Humano Sostenible, Noveno Informe 2002. Ministerio de Planificación Nacional y Política Económica (MIDEPLAN), Sistema de Indicadores sobre Desarrollo Sostenible (SIDES). http://mideplan.go.cr. Date: 09-07-04.

Table 24 **STI´s Obligatory declaration diseases rates 1970, 1975, 1980, 1985, 1990 a 2003 (By 100000 inhabitants)**

Year	Gonorrhea	Siphylis	AIDS
1970*	162.0	56.0	0.0
1975*	143.0	75.0	0.0
1980*	477.0	99.0	0.0
1985*	314.0	57.0	---
1990*	142.0	64.0	3.0
1991*	119.0	41.0	3.0
1992	124.6	56.4	5.2
1993	56.4	30.5	3.9
1994	62.7	35.8	4.9
1995	68.6	44.7	5.9
1996	52.6	37.1	3.4
1997	56.6	41.4	7.1
1998	56.3	36.9	7.5
1999	50.4	23.5	5.7
2000	33.3	20.3	7.0
2001	31.8	19.8	3.5
2002	23.4	18.7	1.0
2003*	55.0	18.0	3.0

Source: Proyecto Estado de la Nación en Desarrollo Humano Sostenible, Noveno Informe 2002. Ministerio de Planificación Nacional y Política Económica (MIDEPLAN), Sistema de Indicadores sobre Desarrollo Sostenible (SIDES). http://mideplan.go.cr. Date: 09-07-04.

Table 25 **Costa Rica. Commercial sex workers, Recommendations to others sex workers to prevent AIDS**

Recommendations		1997 Study	2000 Study
	(N)	(300)	(400)
	Total	100.0	100.0
Use condom with partner or lover			
Yes, spontaneous		57.2	64.8
Yes, with support		20.7	6.3
No		22.1	29.0
Use condom with regular clients			
Yes, spontaneous		87.7	85.5
Yes, with support		8.7	10.8
No		3.7	3.8
Use condom with occasional clients			
Yes, spontaneous		88.0	84.8
Yes, with support		10.4	13.3
No		1.7	2.0
Avoid anal penetration			
Yes, spontaneous		10.0	2.3
Yes, with support		80.3	89.0
No		9.7	8.8
Avoid any type of oral sex			
Yes, spontaneous		7.7	2.0
Yes, with support		35.9	60.0
No		56.4	38.0
Use condom in oral sex			
Yes, spontaneous		12.7	2.0
Yes, with support		71.6	84.0
No		15.7	14.0
Masturbate clients			
Yes, spontaneous		4.4	0.3
Yes, with support		61.7	77.3
No		33.9	22.5

Avoid inside ejaculation			
Yes, spontaneous		5.7	0.8
Yes, with support		82.9	91.0
No		11.4	8.3
Avoid drug and alcohol			
Yes, spontaneous		11.3	1.5
Yes, with support		79.7	87.0
No		9.0	11.5

Table 26 **Costa Rica. Commercial sex workers, Changes made since they heard about AIDS**

Changes		1997 Study	2000 Study
	(N)	(300)	(400)
	Total	100.0	100.0
Use condom with partner or lover			
Yes, spontaneous		29.4	35.3
Yes, with support		6.7	8.0
No		63.9	56.8
Use condom with regular clients			
Yes, spontaneous		77.7	56.8
Yes, with support		11.7	33.5
No		10.7	9.8
Use condom with occasional clients			
Yes, spontaneous		75.7	56.3
Yes, with support		18.3	38.8
No		6.0	5.0
Avoid anal penetration			
Yes, spontaneous		12.0	2.0
Yes, with support		78.3	85.9
No		9.7	12.1

Avoid any type of oral sex		
Yes, spontaneous	9.0	2.5
Yes, with support	38.3	81.5
No	52.7	16.0

Use condom in oral sex		
Yes, spontaneous	9.4	2.5
Yes, with support	68.1	81.5
No	22.5	16.0

Masturbate clients		
Yes, spontaneous	5.7	0.5
Yes, with support	60.0	71.8
No	34.3	27.8

Avoid inside ejaculation		
Yes, spontaneous	6.3	1.3
Yes, with support	79.3	83.5
No	14.3	15.3

Avoid drug and alcohol		
Yes, spontaneous	8.0	1.3
Yes, with support	70.6	82.5
No	21.4	16.3

Index

Page numbers followed by the letter "t" indicates tables.

A

F

G

I

J

K

L

M

P

Q

R

S

T

U

W

About the author

Jacobo Schifter, PhD in History from Columbia University (1983), is Emeritus Profesor at Universidad Nacional in Costa Rica. He has published several controversial books on Costa Rican–US relations and on Costa Rica's Civil War. He has also published several books on AIDS and sexuality, including Lila's House. A Study on Male Prostitution in Latin America (Haworth, 1998), Macho Love. Sex Behind Bars in Latin America (Haworth, 1999), From Toads to Queens. Transvestim in a Latin American Setting, (Haworth, 2000), Public Sex in Latin America (Haworth, 2000), Truckdrivers's Trade (Haworth, 2001).

www.ingramcontent.com/pod-product-compliance
Ingram Content Group UK Ltd.
Pitfield, Milton Keynes, MK11 3LW, UK
UKHW041142300926
15471UKWH00011B/96

9 780761 835974